IMPROVING CARE
FOR VETERANS WITH TRAUMATIC BRAIN INJURY ACROSS THE LIFESPAN

Kathryn E. Bouskill | Carrie M. Farmer | Irineo Cabreros

Jonathan Cantor | Natalie Ernecoff | Lynn Hu | Shira H. Fischer

Aaron Kofner | Lisa S. Meredith | Matthew L. Mizel | Aneesa Motala

Tepring Piquado | Zachary Predmore | Rajeev Ramchand

Sponsored by Wounded Warrior Project

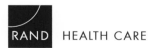

RAND HEALTH CARE

For more information on this publication, visit **www.rand.org/t/RRA1205-1**.

About RAND

The RAND Corporation is a research organization that develops solutions to public policy challenges to help make communities throughout the world safer and more secure, healthier and more prosperous. RAND is nonprofit, nonpartisan, and committed to the public interest. To learn more about RAND, visit www.rand.org.

Research Integrity

Our mission to help improve policy and decisionmaking through research and analysis is enabled through our core values of quality and objectivity and our unwavering commitment to the highest level of integrity and ethical behavior. To help ensure our research and analysis are rigorous, objective, and nonpartisan, we subject our research publications to a robust and exacting quality-assurance process; avoid both the appearance and reality of financial and other conflicts of interest through staff training, project screening, and a policy of mandatory disclosure; and pursue transparency in our research engagements through our commitment to the open publication of our research findings and recommendations, disclosure of the source of funding of published research, and policies to ensure intellectual independence. For more information, visit www.rand.org/about/principles.

Published by the RAND Corporation, Santa Monica, Calif.
© 2022 RAND Corporation
RAND® is a registered trademark.

Library of Congress Cataloging-in-Publication Data is available for this publication.
ISBN: 978-1-9774-0874-7

Cover image courtesy Stacy Pearsall, Veterans Portrait Project

About This Report

Between 2000 and 2021, more than 444,300 service members experienced a traumatic brain injury (TBI) during their military service. There are concerns that those who experienced one or more TBIs may be at higher risk for comorbid health conditions, such as early-onset dementia and premature mortality. As the population of veterans living with TBI continues to increase in both number and age, little is known about the expected course of their condition or how best to meet their needs for long-term support services.

This report describes the findings from a study commissioned by Wounded Warrior Project and conducted by the RAND Corporation to identify the long-term outcomes of TBI for veterans serving since the terrorist attacks of September 11, 2001; the future needs of this population; effective treatments for TBI; and the availability of community-based resources. The information included in this report can be used to better understand which approaches may offer the best care for veterans with TBI, as well as help inform the care and support offered to veterans and their caregivers.

This research was funded by Wounded Warrior Project and carried out within the Quality Measurement and Improvement Program in RAND Health Care.

RAND Health Care, a division of the RAND Corporation, promotes healthier societies by improving health care systems in the United States and other countries. We do this by providing health care decisionmakers, practitioners, and consumers with actionable, rigorous, objective evidence to support their most complex decisions. For more information, see www.rand.org/health-care, or contact

RAND Health Care Communications
1776 Main Street
P.O. Box 2138
Santa Monica, CA 90407-2138
(310) 393-0411, ext. 7775
RAND_Health-Care@rand.org

Acknowledgments

We thank Wounded Warrior Project team members who offered critical support throughout this study, including Alex Balbir, Brian Dempsey, and Lara Berghammer, all of whom were generous with their time, facilitated access to necessary data, and shared information and insights about their programs. We are grateful to the 40 veterans and caregivers, as well as the 15 experts in the field, who shared their experiences and insights with us for this project. We thank Katharine Stout and Andrew Parker, who served as technical peer reviewers. Their feedback helped improve this report. We appreciate Justin Hummer for his contributions to conducting the interviews with subject-matter experts and veterans, as well as Alicia Locker for her work on reviewing the literature in an earlier draft of this report. We thank Kristin Leuschner for writing and editorial assistance. Gabriela Alvarado, Samer Atshan, Jalal Awan, Elliott Brennan, Swaptik Chowdhury, Clark Gardner, Ishita Ghai, Tim Gulden, and Sujeong Park provided essential help with abstracting and cleaning the TBI resources data, while Carlos Calvo Hernandez and Samer Atshan created the visualization based on the resulting data set. Finally, we thank our project assistant, Roshon Gibson, for her efforts to keep the study on track.

Summary

Traumatic brain injury (TBI) is often considered one of the signature injuries of veterans who served in the U.S. military after September 11, 2001 (9/11). Although not all military-related TBIs are recorded, the U.S. Department of Defense (DoD) reports that more than 444,300 service members experienced a TBI between 2000 and 2021 (Corrigan et al., 2020; Military Health System, undated-a; Military Health System, undated-b; Traumatic Brain Injury Center of Excellence, 2021). Veterans with TBI often have co-occurring conditions, such as posttraumatic stress disorder (PTSD), and may be at higher risk for other health conditions, such as early-onset dementia and premature mortality.

Much progress has been made to identify, treat, and manage patients with TBI, but gaps remain in our understanding of the long-term care and support needs of veterans who have sustained one or more TBIs during their military service, especially those who served in the military on or after 9/11. Furthermore, the needs of veterans who have sustained a TBI are not uniform. In addition, the U.S. veteran population is becoming increasingly diverse with respect to race, ethnicity, and gender (Office of Data Governance and Analytics, 2017), and post-9/11 veterans are the most diverse population among all combat eras (National Center for Veterans Analysis and Statistics, 2018). The combination of a diverse and aging population dealing with the long-term impacts of a complex disorder creates challenging questions about the expected course of recovery and how best to provide care and support. Several large, longitudinal research studies funded by DoD, the U.S. Department of Veterans Affairs (VA), and public-private partnerships are underway with the goal of understanding the long-term impacts of TBI and identifying promising treatment approaches. Although these studies will yield important information, organizations serving veterans with TBI need actionable information today to meet and plan for the needs of this population over time.

In response to these concerns, Wounded Warrior Project (WWP) commissioned the RAND Corporation to examine what is known about the long-term outcomes of TBI for post-9/11 veterans, the future needs of this population, effective treatments for TBI, and the availability of community-based supports. As part of that effort, we sought to develop guidance and recommendations for organizations that serve veterans with TBI, including DoD, VA, and WWP, and to help inform future investments and improvements in the care and support of these veterans.

Our mixed methods included a systematic review of systematic reviews (known as an *umbrella review*) to understand long-term outcomes following TBI and treatment options, analysis of data from WWP's Annual Warrior Survey, semi-structured interviews with veterans with TBI and their caregivers, a systematic review of the literature on treatment of long-term outcomes following TBI, identification and classification of existing support and points of care for military-related TBI, and semi-structured interviews with subject-matter experts to identify key challenges and opportunities surrounding the identification of TBI and its treatment over the long term.

What Is Traumatic Brain Injury?

TBI is a serious injury to the head that causes damage to the brain. TBI can result from many causes, including military service, accidents, and engagement in contact sports or risky behaviors. TBIs vary in severity—from mild to moderate and severe—and the severity of a TBI is classified at the time of injury. However, severity of TBI does not necessarily correspond to long-term outcomes. For example, some individuals who experienced a mild TBI (also known as a *concussion*) may have ongoing disability, while someone with a moderate TBI may completely recover.

TBI is considered a hallmark injury among post-9/11 veterans. Most military-related TBIs are considered mild (82 percent); moderate injuries are less common (11 percent); few injuries are considered severe (1 percent) or a result of a penetrating wound (1 percent); and some are not classifiable (5 percent) (Military Health System, undated-a). Military-related TBIs tend to differ from civilian TBIs in several key ways. In particular, improvised explosive devices were one of the leading causes of TBI among veterans who deployed to Iraq and Afghanistan (Perl, 2016). In some cases, blast-related TBIs may initially result in little visible harm, yet widespread neurologic and behavioral symptoms can appear later. Prior to increased TBI surveillance and awareness, TBI was often under-identified and did not always result in medical evacuation or proper treatment (Tanielian and Jaycox, 2008). Although research from sports-related and civilian TBIs may have some applicability to understanding and treating blast injuries, the neurologic effect of primary blast injuries may fundamentally differ from the effect of most sources of civilian TBIs (Warden, 2006).

Because military-related brain injuries are complex, often co-occur with other injuries, and may be compounded by previous TBIs, the course of treatment varies considerably from veteran to veteran. Initial treatment of a moderate to severe TBI generally includes addressing both the head injury and any other injuries until the patient is stabilized. Following initial treatment, veterans may receive physical therapy, occupational therapy, and therapy for cognitive and emotional problems associated with TBI. Most patients with a single mild TBI recover within a few weeks of their injury, although 10 to 20 percent have ongoing symptoms, including *post-concussion syndrome*, a condition characterized by a constellation of cognitive, physical, and psychological symptoms lasting months after a mild TBI (Farmer et al., 2016).

Long-Term Outcomes of Traumatic Brain Injury

Given the large volume of research on TBI, we conducted an umbrella review, as noted earlier, to summarize systematic reviews on the risk or prevalence of long-term outcomes after TBI. Systematic reviews and meta-analyses were eligible for inclusion in this analysis if the population in the included articles was adults with a diagnosed TBI of any severity. We excluded reviews if the population was adults with other types of brain injuries (e.g., brain injuries caused by something other than an external physical force to the head), including stroke. We also excluded reviews of solely pediatric and adolescent populations.

We identified a large number of systematic reviews and meta-analyses that explored the relationship between TBI and long-term outcomes, although the ability to measure changes in long-term outcomes was limited. Systematic reviews examined long-term outcomes after TBI across several domains, including cognitive outcomes, such as memory and attention; physical outcomes, such as headaches and sleep quality; and co-occurring health conditions, such as PTSD, depression, dementia, amyotrophic lateral sclerosis (ALS), and Parkinson's disease. On the whole, the literature suggested that long-term outcomes were worse for TBI patients (compared with patients without TBI) across cognitive domains, although the strength of evidence varied depending on the cognitive domain, the severity of the TBI, and the time since the injury. In addition, evidence suggested that people with TBI had poorer physical long-term outcomes, including the prevalence of pain.

Of all outcome domains, co-occurring psychological conditions and subsequently developed health conditions were the most commonly studied. On the whole, the reviews suggested that TBI was associated with higher risk of a variety of psychological health conditions, although the strength of that relationship varied according to the condition studied. Reviews found mixed evidence for the relationship between TBI and dementia and limited evidence for an association between TBI and other neurodegenerative conditions, such as ALS and Parkinson's disease, and conditions involving pituitary problems. However, these studies reported on relatively rare conditions and may have been limited by recall bias and other problems.

Relatively few reviews reported prevalence of these long-term outcomes, and those that did showed an increased relative risk, often estimated as a small overall absolute risk increase over the long term. Several studies that stratified outcomes by the number of years post-injury even found decreasing odds of negative outcomes with time.

Very few reviews looked at functional, social, or occupational outcomes, which are often important for patients. We also did not identify any reviews that made a quantitative assessment of the impact of TBI on health care costs. Reviews that incorporated weights by evidence quality or that limited analyses to medium- or high-quality evidence found a smaller effect of TBI on negative outcomes. Furthermore, many studies noted that they were not able to establish causation, especially for PTSD, which may be caused by an unobserved confounding variable that also caused the TBI (e.g., blast trauma). Very few reviews included only veteran populations, and, given the unique experiences and needs of this population, the applicability of reviews focusing on TBI among athletes or the general adult population may be limited.

In addition, very few reviews (less than 20 percent) accounted for gender when assessing TBI outcomes, indicating that future research into TBI outcomes should take gender into account. Even fewer reviews looked at outcomes by race or ethnicity, suggesting another important area for future research.

Many reviews were also relatively inconsistent in the length of follow-up in the included studies. The follow-up in these included studies often ranged from one to ten or more years. About half of the reviews included TBI of all severity levels (mild, moderate, and severe), and some studies focused only on mild TBI or concussion or only on severe TBI.

Characteristics of WWP Alumni with Traumatic Brain Injury and Other Head Injuries

The WWP Annual Warrior Survey is a rich source of information for identifying characteristics and potential needs of subpopulations, including veterans who experienced head injuries.[1] Survey responses provide a data-driven approach to ensure that WWP is serving the populations that it intends to serve and to help WWP learn about what additional services it can provide to meet those populations' needs. In addition, the survey helps identify how subpopulations differ from one another so that WWP can learn whether there are unique needs or gaps that need to be addressed. We received three years (2017, 2018, 2020) of survey data from WWP for our analysis.

The analysis revealed many differences between veterans who had experienced a head injury and those who had not. For example, relative to those without a head injury, those in the group who self-reported having sustained a head injury during their military service were more likely to be men, more likely to have retired from the service for medical reasons, and more likely to have served in the Army and Marine Corps. They also tended to be more severely impaired and to have higher disability ratings from VA and the DoD Physical Evaluation Board, more comorbidities, and a greater reliance on caregivers. Although veterans with a head injury were less likely to be employed, comparable proportions of those with and without a head injury were enrolled in school; still, a greater proportion of enrollees with a head injury were using government assistance to finance their education.

We found that, after controlling for multiple factors, veterans with a head injury were more likely to report elevated PTSD and depression symptoms.[2] Surprisingly, after controlling for such factors as physical and mental injuries and the need for caregiver support, those with a head injury had better self-reported health. There was no association between having a head injury and sleep quality after model adjustment.

Although WWP alumni with a head injury were more likely to have VA health insurance and Medicare and more likely to have recently used medical and mental health care, they still faced multiple challenges in accessing care, including breaks in the continuity of care and difficulty scheduling appointments. Other challenges included distrust of government-sponsored services and lack of available specialized VA services. Although veterans with a head injury reported greater need for services across multiple domains than those without did, the use of WWP programs and services was roughly comparable between the two groups.

---

[1] We use the term *veterans* when describing WWP survey results but acknowledge that some *alumni* (the term WWP uses to refer to the service members and veterans who receive its services) are still serving in the military.

[2] Survey respondents were asked to "choose all that apply" to indicate "any severe physical or mental injuries or health problems you experienced while serving, or as a result of serving, in the military after September 11, 2001." Response options included "traumatic brain injury (TBI)" and "head injuries other than traumatic brain injury (TBI)."

Long-Term Experiences of Traumatic Brain Injury Among Veterans and Caregivers

WWP identified alumni who, in 2011 or earlier, self-reported a TBI with the program, and WWP then sent an email to those individuals with a request to participate in an interview regarding their experiences living with TBI. Veterans could express interest in participating in an interview by calling or emailing the RAND team or by signing up on a RAND website. Veterans were invited to ask their caregivers, if applicable, to participate in a separate interview about the caregiver's own experience. Caregivers were also able to reach out to RAND independently of the veteran for whom they provide care.

The sample of veterans who volunteered to participate in an interview skewed toward those with more-moderate or more-severe TBI, which may explain why the majority of veterans in the sample reported enduring serious challenges. Complications in treating their TBI began in the combat zone, where some then–service members were reluctant or unable to seek care for TBI. As a result, many veterans reported sustaining several TBIs before suffering one definitive blow that was accompanied by other physical injuries. Interviewees explained that receiving a diagnosis and timely treatment was not straightforward, and many described seeking treatment for many years in several locations offering varying degrees of care. Veterans' search for care and perceived success with treatment were further complicated by comorbid conditions, especially PTSD, migraines, and cognitive challenges, which were pervasive across this sample of veterans.

The cognitive challenges that many veterans expressed difficulty with included remembering what to get from the grocery store and following a conversation. Such challenges have taken a major toll on veterans' identities, their ability to seek employment and pursue education, their romantic relationships, and the well-being of their families, as confirmed by their caregivers. Several veterans described coping with these challenges by providing service to others, particularly other veterans.

It is important to note that this qualitative analysis focused on veterans who were injured several years prior to the interview and that both basic science and clinical research on TBI, as well as delivery of health services, have made important strides in recent years. These experiences may not reflect those of veterans who were treated more recently or those who did not volunteer to participate in an interview. That being said, clinicians and researchers cannot lose sight of the needs of the aging veterans who did not have access to newer treatments and may therefore be facing additional challenges and service needs.

Looking to the future, the veterans in this sample were concerned about accelerated aging and early-onset dementia. They were looking for answers and ways to prepare for the physical and cognitive challenges that they were facing. The veterans were proactively working through their reported limitations and leveraging their resources to establish a new normal.

Treatments and Interventions to Address Long-Term Outcomes from Traumatic Brain Injury

The systematic reviews that we identified assessed diverse types of interventions, including to support those with TBI; those interventions include pharmaco- and psychotherapy, rehabilitation, brain stimulation, hyperbaric oxygen therapy, and complementary and alternative medicine. Regarding the effectiveness of different interventions, evidence supports cognitive rehabilitation for cognitive outcomes, psychotherapy for psychological outcomes, behavioral interventions for social outcomes, occupational rehabilitation for occupational outcomes, and psychotherapy and behavioral interventions for post-concussion syndrome.

A challenge in understanding the effectiveness of interventions is that most TBI research examines effects on the general adult population and often includes non-TBI neurological diagnoses that may result in imprecise or inaccurate efficacy of interventions to support veterans with TBI specifically. Some studies have incorporated caregivers into interventions, while others are testing promising technological platforms to improve caregiver-facing education and support interventions.

Innovations and traditional treatments for TBI show promise. For example, although evidence is in the early stages, existing studies show that virtual reality may support motor and cognitive function (Cano Porras et al., 2018). More broadly, digital approaches to care, including telehealth, may improve access and resources for people who have mobility or functional limitations or comorbidities, who are homebound, or who live far from traditional care and rehabilitation centers (Zhou and Parmanto, 2019). However, additional high-quality research in veteran populations is essential to understanding the most-effective interventions for improving outcomes after TBI.

Resources Available to Veterans with Traumatic Brain Injury

Several specialty care facilities and treatment centers have been established to address the unique needs of veterans with TBI. These include the National Intrepid Center of Excellence at the Walter Reed National Military Medical Center in Bethesda, Maryland; the Marcus Institute for Brain Health at the University of Colorado Anschutz Medical Campus in Aurora, Colorado; and the SHARE Military Initiative at Shephard Center in Atlanta, Georgia. WWP also established several programs to facilitate access to care and support for post-9/11 veterans living with TBI. These include (1) the Independence Program, a long-term, community-based support program, and (2) the Warrior Care Network, a partnership between WWP and four academic medical centers to provide intensive outpatient, evidence-based treatment to veterans with TBI, PTSD, and related conditions. Despite these extensive efforts, access to state-of-the-art TBI care is not universal.

Through a searching and screening process, we identified 2,325 TBI resources across the United States. These resources include medical facilities and other organizations that serve veterans with TBI by providing physical health care, mental health care, and targeted services needed for TBI rehabilitation. We found that the average drive time to a TBI resource was about 30 minutes for WWP alumni, although this depended on the type of resource. For example, WWP alumni typically had faster geographic access to physical health services than to mental health services.

Although our analyses of these data offer insights into geographic access for WWP alumni with TBI, there are some limitations. First, although there are about 6,000 hospitals in the United States, and most have some TBI services, there are 586 hospitals in our database, including all VA medical centers and other hospitals that came up in a search for TBI. We did not include the numerous VA clinics that may offer support for TBI or redirect individuals to other TBI care. Second, we calculated each of the minimum drive time distances using the centroid of the WWP veteran's zip code. Future work should perform similar analyses using the household address of WWP veterans, if possible. This would give a more accurate representation of geographic access because some zip codes cover a large geographic area. Third, although we calculated geographic access to resources, we did not assess the capacity of those resources. Finally, although we calculated the minimum distance to a TBI resource, we did not capture other measures that would affect access, such as what forms of insurance are accepted.

Despite these limitations, we identified a variety of resources across the United States that serve veterans and that focus on TBI needs. We were also able to map locations where services are clustered and where they are lacking, which enabled us to identify potential gaps in access.

Perspectives on Addressing the Long-Term Impacts of Traumatic Brain Injury Among Veterans

Subject-matter experts offered valuable insights into the complex fields of treating and researching TBI. Experts reiterated the complexities of providing a timely diagnosis of TBI and pinning down its severity. In addition, they said that those who sustained a TBI in the early years of the Iraq and Afghanistan wars may not have been readily diagnosed, because regular screening was mandated only after 2007.

Clinicians and researchers noted that experiencing TBI presents an increased risk, albeit modest, for several disorders. Although there were disagreements over the magnitude of this risk, all experts agreed that confounding comorbid conditions (e.g., PTSD) and ambiguity over the number and severity of TBIs make it nearly impossible to make definitive statements about risk for downstream health issues or the best ways to address or mitigate risk for these health issues. All of these experts reinforced the importance of promoting wellness and active engagement in care not only for TBI but also for common comorbid conditions, such as PTSD.

Furthermore, experts described several areas that could advance the state of the science and delivery of care for veterans who sustained a TBI. Across the board, they underscored the need to address limitations in data on veterans with TBI. Those limitations could be mitigated by better syncing data systems across DoD and the Veterans Health Administration, as well as by tracking veterans more concertedly and longitudinally. The experts also described a need for more collaboration across different research camps within TBI and for closer research efforts to understand the links between TBI and PTSD. Enhancing brain banks would also likely advance understanding of key issues surrounding TBI and brain health. Where possible, employing telehealth technologies, which was swiftly expanded during the coronavirus disease 2019 pandemic, could further close gaps in accessing care.

Recommendations

Our findings point to several recommendations for improving care and support for veterans with TBI. These recommendations are intended to guide policymakers, health care systems, veteran-serving organizations, and researchers in their work to improve the long-term outcomes for veterans with TBI and to provide adequate support to their caregivers and families.

Our first set of recommendations center on the need to **create long-term systems of support** for veterans and caregivers:

- **Provide support to veterans and caregivers for long-term planning and expectation-setting.** The narrative accounts of veterans with TBI who participated in this study revealed the challenges of enduring a TBI (or multiple TBIs) and that veterans and caregivers were left with many unanswered questions about what they can expect as veterans age. Veterans and their caregivers should have support for long-term planning and solid case management to manage TBI and complex polytraumas.
- **Increase caregiver support.** Formal long-term options for care are incomplete, and a large amount of the support for veterans with TBI is often left to their informal family caregivers. Veteran-specific resources for long-term care are essential. VA's Program of Comprehensive Assistance for Family Caregivers provides support to caregivers of eligible veterans, but more needs to be done to spread the word about the availability of this program and to reduce barriers to receiving support. In addition, as caregivers themselves age and have reduced capacity to care for their veterans, this VA program may need additional resources and an expanded mission.
- **Expand access to long-term care.** VA does not currently pay for room and board in assisted-living facilities; however, given the expected long-term care needs of veterans with TBI, this policy may need to be reconsidered. VA piloted an assisted-living program for veterans with TBI from 2009 to 2018, which could serve as a model for the future. However, VA may need additional regulatory authority to pay the full cost of long-term rehabilitation, or veterans needing such care may be warranted a supplementary disability benefit to help pay for these costs.

Second, **expand access to multidisciplinary treatment.** Given the co-occurrence of TBI and PTSD, co-locating TBI and PTSD care and research may better serve populations of veterans by delivering culturally appropriate, holistic care. To that end, expanding awareness of the existing programs and care models that provide integrated treatment of these conditions should be prioritized. In addition, it is important to expand access to tailored, multifaceted, and comprehensive treatment, either by incorporating more telehealth and other technology or by widely disseminating best practices.

Third, **promote health-enhancing behaviors.** Health care providers should encourage fundamental wellness—a healthy diet, regular exercise, mindfulness, and abstinence from alcohol and other substances—as a key part of treatment. Participation in health-promoting activities could also serve a critical social function for veterans with TBI and their caregivers, given the importance of forming personal connections with other veterans and families who understand their challenges and with whom they can share a common bond.

Fourth, improving the ability to address the long-term needs of veterans with TBI requires that organizations continue to **collect and integrate better-quality data.**

- **Integrate data on TBI and related conditions across record systems.** In the next five to ten years, DoD and VA are expected to integrate their electronic health records. But until that system comes online, individual-level health, health care, and service history data from DoD and VA could be merged to allow a longitudinal analysis of veterans with TBI. This type of analysis could provide, among other things, new insights into the relationships among the timing of TBI diagnosis and treatment, the types of treatment received, and long-term outcomes.
- **Enhance the WWP Annual Warrior Survey.** WWP should consider creating a longitudinal data file across survey years to track veterans over time. WWP could also consider additional surveys among subpopulations identified in the Annual Warrior Survey, including alumni with a head injury. The goals of these surveys would be to collect more-detailed and tailored information about barriers and challenges that WWP alumni face in accessing health, education, employment, and even WWP programs and services.

Finally, organizations must continue to **invest in research.** Our findings indicate both continued demand and need for high-quality research examining veterans with TBI and corresponding treatments and outcomes. Several treatments, including those facilitated by technology and virtual care, show promise for improving outcomes associated with TBI, but there is not yet sufficient evidence for widespread application, especially in veteran populations. Expanding telehealth interventions and their rigorous evaluation could also be an important means of closing gaps in accessing care within the veteran population, particularly for veterans living in rural regions and those who are not able to reach TBI-specific treatment centers.

- **Conduct longitudinal studies examining variation in outcomes and across different populations.** Veterans with TBI differ in important ways from the general adult population; the cause of injury is one of the most important differences, especially when the TBI is combat-related. A better understanding of the long-term outcomes for veterans with TBI—as well as the intersection among veteran status, race, and gender and how this contributes to access to treatment and outcomes—is critical to improving care for this most diverse population of veterans in the history of the U.S. military.

- **Conduct studies on evidence-based treatments, including holistic treatments, for TBI.** The complexity of TBI and its pervasive, lasting, and differing effects contribute to the gaps in literature on treating TBI. This gap in treatment research may improve when the longer-term effects of TBI are better understood and a greater variety of treatment options are available, including promising treatments that can be used at home or through technology.
- **Expand basic science research.** In our interviews, researchers underscored the advantages that would be conveyed to the field of TBI studies if there were reliable biomarkers for TBI severity and chronic traumatic encephalopathy. Although efforts in this space are well underway, advancing this research could make a significant contribution to *in vivo* diagnostics and more-timely treatment.

Closing Thoughts

WWP, DoD, VA, veterans, and caregivers have all raised concerns about the long-term consequences of military-related TBI. In particular, they are concerned about the risk for early-onset neurodegenerative disorders in an already vulnerable population. The recommendations put forth in this report could help ensure that veterans who served and made significant sacrifices for the United States do not fall through the cracks. Implementing these recommendations will require a collaborative approach among veteran-serving organizations, VA, DoD, and other federal policymakers to ensure that veterans with TBI receive evidence-based treatments and interventions over the long term, along with support and resources for them and their caregivers as they age.

Contents

Figures and Tables

Figures

Tables

CHAPTER ONE

Introduction

Traumatic brain injury (TBI) is often considered to be one of the signature injuries of veterans who served in the military after September 11, 2001 (9/11). Estimates suggest that up to 25 percent of individuals who deployed in support of the wars in Iraq and Afghanistan likely have had a TBI (Lindquist, Love, and Elbogen, 2017). Although not all military-related TBIs are recorded, the U.S. Department of Defense (DoD) reports that more than 444,300 service members experienced a TBI between 2000 and 2021 (Corrigan et al., 2020; Military Health System, undated-a; Military Health System, undated-b; Traumatic Brain Injury Center of Excellence, 2021). Although some veterans with TBI recover completely, many have ongoing challenges related to their TBI. In addition, veterans with TBI often have co-occurring conditions, such as posttraumatic stress disorder (PTSD), and may be at higher risk for other health conditions, such as early-onset dementia and premature mortality.

Significant investments have been made to identify, treat, and manage patients with TBI. This work has included several federal and private-sector efforts to study TBI, create treatment guidelines, and implement new programs and policies. But, although progress has been made toward developing, implementing, and disseminating effective treatments for TBI, significant gaps remain in our understanding of the long-term care and support needs of veterans who sustained one or more TBIs during their military service, especially those who served in the military after 9/11. Furthermore, the needs of veterans who have sustained a TBI are not uniform. TBI does not lend itself to a clear-cut diagnosis, level of severity, and impact on an individual; the same event could create different injuries and symptoms in different individuals. *TBI* is a general term that describes a variety of brain injuries. In addition, the U.S. veteran population is becoming increasingly diverse with respect to race, ethnicity, and gender (Office of Data Governance and Analytics, 2017), and post-9/11 veterans are the most diverse population among all combat eras (National Center for Veterans Analysis and Statistics, 2018). And there are concerns that U.S. special operations forces may suffer from *operator syndrome*—the interrelated difficulties of TBI, endocrine dysfunction, poor sleep hygiene, chronic pain, headaches, substance use, mental health issues, relationship issues, and cognitive impairments (Frueh et al., 2020). The combination of a diverse and aging population dealing with the long-term impacts of a complex disorder creates challenging questions about the expected course of recovery and how best to provide care and support.

In response to these concerns, Wounded Warrior Project (WWP) commissioned the RAND Corporation to conduct a study designed to identify the long-term outcomes of TBI for post-9/11 veterans, the future needs of this population, effective treatments for TBI, and the availability of community-based supports. As part of that effort, we sought to develop guidance and recommendations for organizations that serve veterans with TBI, including the U.S. Department of Veterans Affairs (VA), DoD, and WWP, and to help inform future investments and improvements in the care and support of these veterans.

In the remainder of this chapter, we provide additional background on TBI and offer a brief overview of the research approach used in this study.

What Is Traumatic Brain Injury?

TBI is a serious injury to the head that causes damage to the brain. TBI can result from many causes, including engagement in contact sports, risky behaviors, or dangerous lifestyles. One of the risk factors for TBI is military service, where service members are regularly exposed to combat situations and high-powered firearm use and are at increased risk for blast injuries (Kim and Gean, 2011).

TBIs vary in severity—from mild to moderate and severe—and the severity of a TBI is classified at the time of injury. TBIs that involve penetration to the brain are referred to as *penetrating brain injuries.* Closed head injuries resulting from blunt force trauma (e.g., exposure to a blast, impact from falls) may be further classified along a continuum—mild, moderate, or severe—based on five indexes (Table 1.1). Severity of TBI does not necessarily correspond to long-term outcomes, however. For example, some individuals who experienced a mild TBI (also known as a *concussion*) may have ongoing disability, while someone with a moderate TBI may completely recover.

Although many people recover from a single TBI, especially if it is mild, service members are more likely than civilians to be exposed to multiple TBIs and have unique causes of injury, such as a large-scale explosive blast. A TBI of any severity can produce changes in the

TABLE 1.1
Traumatic Brain Injury Severity Criteria

Index	Mild	Moderate	Severe
Structural imaging	Normal	Normal or abnormal	Normal or abnormal
Loss of consciousness	0–30 minutes	> 30 minutes and < 24 hours	> 24 hours
Alteration of consciousness	Up to 24 hours	> 24 hours; severity based on the other criteria in this table	> 24 hours; severity based on the other criteria in this table
Posttraumatic amnesia	0–1 day	> 1 day and < 7 days	> 7 days
Glasgow Coma Scale score	13–15	9–12	> 9

SOURCE: VA and DoD, 2021.

brain and biological responses in the central nervous system and other parts of the body. The regions of the brain affected by large-scale blasts or repetitive subconcussive head injuries are often those involved with high-level brain functioning tasks, such as decisionmaking, rational thought, emotional inhibition, and memory processing and storage (McAllister, 2011). The biological consequences of TBI may lead to secondary effects, including behavioral, cognitive, and functional issues. But, as noted earlier, the long-term effects of having a military-related TBI are not well understood. Some researchers and clinicians have raised concerns that TBI may be associated with Alzheimer's disease or other dementias, while others feel that the evidence is too inconclusive to make this claim.

Military-Related Traumatic Brain Injury

Most military-related TBIs are considered mild (82 percent), while moderate injuries are less common (11 percent) (Military Health System, undated-a). Few injuries are considered severe (1 percent) or a result of a penetrating wound (1 percent), and 5 percent are not classifiable. Certain characteristics are associated with increased risk for military-related TBI (e.g., male gender, enlisted rank, combat exposure, multiple deployments), and the odds of experiencing a TBI double if a service member has experienced a previous head injury (Lindquist, Love, and Elbogen, 2017; Wilk et al., 2012). RAND's 2008 *Invisible Wounds of War* study indicated that 20 percent of veterans who served in Iraq and Afghanistan reported having experienced a TBI (Tanielian and Jaycox, 2008). Additional research supports this estimate: Studies of Army combat brigades serving in Iraq indicated that 15 to 23 percent of soldiers had sustained a TBI (Hoge et al., 2008; Terrio et al., 2009). By one report, about half of veterans with TBI who served in Iraq or Afghanistan had experienced multiple head injuries (Lindquist, Love, and Elbogen, 2017). Additionally, many service members sustain mild TBI before their time in the military, enhancing the detrimental effects of TBIs during their service (Bryan and Clemans, 2013). The proportion of TBIs that result in long-term effects remains unclear (Chapman and Diaz-Arrastia, 2014).

Military-related TBIs tend to differ from civilian TBIs in several key ways. In particular, improvised explosive devices (IEDs) were one of the leading causes of TBI among veterans who deployed to Iraq and Afghanistan (Perl, 2016). Modern protective equipment has allowed service members to survive such blast injuries, although the resulting brain injury can be severe. In some cases, blast-related TBIs may initially result in little visible harm, yet widespread neurologic and behavioral symptoms can appear later. Prior to increased TBI surveillance and awareness, TBI was often under-identified and did not always result in medical evacuation or proper treatment (Tanielian and Jaycox, 2008). Although research from sports-related and civilian TBIs may have some applicability to understanding and treating blast injuries, the neurologic effect of primary blast injuries may fundamentally differ from the effect of most sources of civilian TBIs (Warden, 2006).

Treatment of Traumatic Brain Injury Among Veterans

Because military-related brain injuries are complex, often co-occur with other injuries, and may be compounded by previous TBIs, the course of treatment varies considerably from veteran to veteran. Initial treatment of a moderate to severe TBI generally includes addressing both the head injury and any other injuries until the patient is stabilized. Following initial treatment, veterans may receive physical therapy, occupational therapy, and therapy for cognitive and emotional problems associated with TBI. Veterans who are enrolled in VA health care and who have more-severe TBI and associated disabilities with a likelihood of returning to independent living may receive care through one of five VA facilities that offer Polytrauma Transitional Rehabilitation Programs (VA, undated-a; undated-c). If deployed overseas at the time of injury, these veterans would have been evacuated to a larger base or, if medically stable, back to the United States for treatment.

Most patients with a single mild TBI recover within a few weeks of their injury, although 10 to 20 percent have ongoing symptoms, including *post-concussion syndrome* (PCS), a condition characterized by a constellation of cognitive, physical, and psychological symptoms lasting months after a mild TBI (Farmer et al., 2016). Veterans who sustain a mild TBI during their military service likely receive initial care from DoD's military health system through on-base services provided at military treatment facilities and clinics; through civilian network providers; or, if deployed, from a field medical hospital. If ongoing treatment is required, veterans with mild TBI may receive care from VA, TRICARE (the health care program for active-duty service members, their families, and military retirees), or the private sector (e.g., through private insurance).

Specialty Treatment Programs for Veterans

Several specialty care facilities and treatment centers have been established to address the unique needs of veterans with TBI. For example, the National Intrepid Center of Excellence at the Walter Reed National Military Medical Center in Bethesda, Maryland, provides a four-week intensive outpatient program for service members with TBI to develop a tailored treatment plan. The center has helped develop TBI standards of care that are used throughout the Military Health System. In addition, the Marcus Institute for Brain Health at the University of Colorado Anschutz Medical Campus in Aurora, Colorado, and the SHARE Military Initiative at Shephard Center in Atlanta, Georgia, provide intensive outpatient treatment to veterans with TBI at no cost to the veteran. These two programs provide multidisciplinary evaluation and treatment and coordinate post-program care with veterans' treatment providers at home. They are both part of the Gary Sinise Foundation's Avalon Network, which was established in 2021 with plans to develop additional treatment sites across the country.

WWP established several programs designed to facilitate access to care and support for post-9/11 veterans living with TBI. For instance, the Independence Program is a long-term, community-based support program for those living with moderate to severe TBI, spinal cord injury, or other neurological conditions. The program pairs post-9/11 veterans and their caregivers with specialized case management teams to help develop personalized plans to restore meaningful levels of activity, purpose, and independence into their daily lives. The Warrior Care Network is a partnership between WWP and four academic medical centers (Emory Healthcare, Massachusetts General Hospital, Rush University Medical Center, and UCLA Health). Warrior Care Network sites provide intensive outpatient, evidence-based treatment to veterans with TBI, PTSD, and related conditions at no cost to the veteran.

Long-Term Care

Currently, VA provides long-term care primarily in nursing homes and through home health care (Bagalman, 2015). Eligible veterans (i.e., those who require 24-hour supervision and assistance with activities of daily living) can receive nursing home care in VA community living centers and non-VA nursing homes. Veterans may also be able to receive nursing home care from State Veterans Homes, which are owned and managed by states. Some veterans may be eligible for VA Medical Foster Homes, in which a veteran lives in a private home and receives care from a trained caregiver. In addition, through its Traumatic Brain Injury – Residential Rehabilitation program, VA provides residential rehabilitation to veterans with TBI whose needs cannot be met by a nursing home or other setting of care (VA, 2021). And VA provides eligible veterans with home-based primary care and other home health care, such as a home health aide. In general, veterans are eligible for these services based on their service-connected status, level of disability, and income and may need to pay for part of this care through other insurance or out of pocket.

Long-Term Needs of Veterans with Traumatic Brain Injury

Although the severity of TBI at the time of the injury is useful for predicting outcomes, there is still wide variation in the long-term trajectory of symptom improvement following injury (Novack et al., 2001). Among those with a moderate or severe TBI, the long-term outcomes may span full recovery to relying completely on others for care and assistance with daily functioning. Significant cognitive and physical functioning deficits often remain even a year post-injury (Andelic et al., 2018; Novack et al., 2000). Alternatively, for most patients with a single mild TBI, the majority of symptoms tend to resolve within weeks after the injury (McCrea et al., 2009), and cognitive symptoms largely subside after three months. However, for some people, symptoms and cognitive deficits may continue unresolved for years (Ruff, 2005), and those with multiple TBIs have worse outcomes (Merritt et al., 2020), including higher risk for suicide (Bryan and Clemans, 2013).

People diagnosed with TBI often have other, comorbid conditions (Pugh et al., 2016). These conditions are not only varied but also pervasive: TBI is linked to a variety of outcomes that appear in all aspects of life, from physical ailments to social and relationship outcomes. For example, TBI can co-occur with mental health and substance use disorders (Adams, Corrigan, and Larson, 2012; Bjork and Grant, 2009; Corrigan and Mysiw, 2012). Because the event that causes TBI can also cause PTSD, veterans sometimes turn to substance use to cope with the symptoms of these conditions, which can contribute to alcohol abuse or other substance use disorders (Weil, Corrigan, and Karelina, 2018). Thus, TBI is frequently wrapped up in a constellation of synergistic disorders, and treatment to address it occurs within a complex system of care.

Ongoing Research Studies

How veterans with TBI fare over the years and decades following their injury remains an important question. The overwhelming research focus to date has been on addressing TBI immediately following an injury. More recently, concerns have been raised regarding the long-term impacts of TBI on the functioning, physical and mental health, and well-being of veterans. In particular, some researchers have raised concerns that TBI is linked to early-onset dementia, chronic traumatic encephalopathy (CTE) (Pattinson and Gill, 2018), Alzheimer's disease (LoBue et al., 2018), and Parkinson's disease (Gardner et al., 2018).

Several recent and ongoing research studies are making significant contributions to the knowledge base by exploring the long-term impacts of TBI on functioning and well-being and identifying novel treatment and prevention approaches. For example, the Defense Health Agency's Traumatic Brain Injury Center of Excellence conducts clinical research on brain injuries across a network of military treatment facilities and VA medical centers. In fulfillment of the 2007 congressional mandate to conduct longitudinal research on the effects of TBI on service members who served in Iraq and Afghanistan, the center is conducting three large-scale, longitudinal studies collectively known as the 15-year studies, which will be complete in 2025 (Traumatic Brain Injury Center of Excellence, 2021). The center also manages a portfolio of congressionally mandated research on blast injuries. To further these efforts, the Defense Health Agency implemented the Warfighter Brain Health Initiative and Strategy in 2020. The initiative aims to advance brain science, with a focus on prevention, TBI exposure, and the long-term effects of TBI (Lee, Khatri, and Fudge, 2020).

As a complement to the DoD studies, VA conducts several large-scale TBI studies, including the Improved Understanding of Medical and Psychological Needs in Service Members and Veterans with Chronic Traumatic Brain Injury study, which examines the rehabilitation and health care needs of service members and veterans with TBI. Other notable VA studies related to TBI include the following:

- The Million Veteran Program is a VA initiative to amass clinical and genetic data across a variety of disorders, including TBI, that affect veterans. Current TBI-related studies focus on biological and genetic markers associated with neurobehavioral and neuropsychological outcomes of TBI (VA, undated-b).
- The Translational Research Center for TBI and Stress Disorders (TRACTS) at the Boston VA is a Rehabilitation Research and Development National Center established to identify the unique needs of post-9/11 veterans with deployment-related TBI and PTSD (Translational Research Center for TBI and Stress Disorders, 2021).

- VA, Boston University, and the Concussion Legacy Foundation maintain a large-scale brain tissue repository to identify diagnostic risk factors, develop a test for CTE, and better understand the long-term impacts of mild TBI and CTE (Boston University CTE Center, undated).

Several research consortia are also examining the long-term impacts of and potential treatments for TBI among veterans and service members. Examples of such consortia include the following:

- The Long-Term Impact of Military-Relevant Brain Injury Consortium – Chronic Effects of Neurotrauma Consortium (LIMBIC-CENC) has conducted a prospective, longitudinal study of mild TBI since 2013. A public-private consortium, the organization was initiated in response to a 2012 executive order to improve the prevention, diagnosis, and treatment of mild TBI (Long-Term Impact of Military-Relevant Brain Injury Consortium – Chronic Effects of Neurotrauma Consortium, undated).
- The National Collegiate Athletic Association and DoD teamed up to establish the Concussion Assessment, Research, and Education (CARE) Consortium in 2014. This has become a large-scale initiative to study the clinical presentation and neurobiological impacts of concussion and repetitive head impact among student-athletes and military service members (National Collegiate Athletic Association, undated).
- The Transforming Research and Clinical Knowledge in Traumatic Brain Injury (TRACK-TBI) study is a multicenter, public-private partnership to generate a precision medicine data set on TBI across civilian, athlete, and military populations. The researchers seek to identify diagnostic and prognostic markers in order to create more-precise assessments of TBI outcomes (Transforming Research and Clinical Knowledge in TBI, undated).

Finally, in early 2021, the National Academies of Science, Engineering, and Medicine initiated the Accelerating Progress in Traumatic Brain Injury Research and Care study, bringing together a committee of experts to develop a ten-year roadmap for research and clinical care for TBI. The final report for that study had not yet been released at the time of writing this report.

Overview of This Study

Although there is a plethora of ongoing research to understand the long-term impacts of TBI and the needs of veterans and their families, organizations serving veterans with TBI need actionable information today to meet and plan for the needs of this population over time. This report provides a synthesis of existing research; qualitative analysis of the on-the-ground realities for veterans with TBI and their caregivers, as well as challenges and opportunities in the clinical and research communities; and recommendations about the types of programs, research, and support that veterans with TBI may need over time. To conduct this study, we carried out six main tasks:

1. We conducted a systematic review of systematic reviews (also known as an *umbrella review*) to describe the research on long-term outcomes following TBI.
2. We analyzed data from WWP's Annual Warrior Survey to understand the differences in employment, other physical and mental health conditions, and other outcomes between WWP alumni with and without a self-reported head injury from military service.
3. Through semi-structured interviews, we elicited veteran and caregiver perspectives about living with or caring for someone with TBI.
4. We conducted a systematic review of the literature on treatment of long-term outcomes following TBI and developed an evidence map to describe the state of the evidence and identify research gaps.
5. We identified and classified existing support and points of care for military-related TBI and developed a database of these resources. This database was geocoded by zip code to facilitate searching these resources by local area.
6. Through semi-structured interviews, we elicited the perspectives of subject-matter experts to identify key challenges and opportunities surrounding the identification of TBI and its treatment over the long term.

These tasks are described in more detail in the relevant chapters.

Organization of This Report

With this report, we seek to expand the understanding of TBI and identify potential strategies for improving outcomes and increasing access to evidence-based care for veterans with TBI across the lifespan. In the following chapters, we summarize the findings from the six tasks described in the previous section. These interrelated components include literature reviews, secondary data analysis, interviews, and resource mapping. In Chapter Two, we report the findings from the umbrella review on long-term health and well-being outcomes. In Chapter Three, we present the results from analysis of data on characteristics of WWP alumni with TBI. In Chapter Four, we present the results from interviews with veterans and caregivers. In Chapter Five, we present findings from the evidence map to identify treatments and interventions for addressing long-term outcomes for veterans with TBI. In Chapter Six, we present results from the landscape analysis of resources for those with TBI. In Chapter Seven, we report on the perspectives of subject-matter experts on addressing the long-term impacts of TBI among veterans. In Chapter Eight, we provide an overall discussion with recommendations for how to allocate resources with the goal of improving TBI care over the course of veterans' lives. In a set of appendixes, we provide search terms and additional data analyses.

CHAPTER TWO

Long-Term Health and Well-Being Outcomes

As described in the previous chapter, the catalyst for this report was to better understand the long-term outcomes for veterans who experienced a TBI. In this chapter, we report the results from our systematic umbrella literature review examining the effects of TBI on a variety of outcomes. We start by describing our search and review approach, then discuss the specific outcomes reported in the systematic reviews included, and finally summarize the findings across all of these reviews. We also report on the limitations of both the systematic reviews and the underlying studies.

Approach to the Umbrella Review of Long-Term Outcomes Following Traumatic Brain Injury

Given the large volume of research on TBI, we conducted a systematic review of systematic reviews, also known as an umbrella review, to summarize the research literature on the risk or prevalence of long-term outcomes after TBI. We began by developing a set of search terms for four databases that are widely used to index relevant research: PubMed, PsycInfo, Web of Science, and PROSPERO (the International Prospective Register of Systematic Reviews). Search terms are included in Appendix A.

Eligibility Criteria

Eligibility criteria were defined using the following PICOTSS (population, intervention, comparators, outcomes, timing, setting, and study design) framework:

- *Population:* Systematic reviews and meta-analyses were eligible for inclusion if the populations in included articles were adult humans with a diagnosed TBI of any severity. We excluded reviews if the population was adults with other types of brain injuries (e.g., brain injuries caused by something other than an external physical force to the head), including stroke. We also excluded reviews of solely pediatric and adolescent populations.
- *Intervention:* We excluded reviews that solely evaluated interventions (see Chapter Five for a review of interventions). We excluded TBI case series or reviews of clinical case reports.

- *Comparators:* Reviews were not restricted by comparator.
- *Outcomes:* We included systematic reviews that broadly assessed long-term outcomes associated with TBI, which we defined as outcomes more than a year post-injury. Reviews were eligible for inclusion if they reported on outcomes less than a year after the injury if they also included outcomes more than a year after the injury.
- *Timing:* We did not restrict based on publication year.
- *Setting:* We did not restrict based on setting. We did not restrict based on language.
- *Study design:* We included systematic reviews. Included reviews reported the prevalence, relative risk, or odds ratios associated with outcomes of TBI. We also included reviews that produced narrative syntheses. We excluded reviews that assessed the impact of only a comorbidity or predictor on outcomes for TBI patients.

Data Extraction

We developed a data extraction form to collect relevant information from included reviews. This form included fields about the design of the review (number of databases searched, number of included reviews, date of last search). We categorized participants into three groups: veterans, athletes, and the general adult population. We also collected information about the conditions and outcomes in the review, as well as any limitations noted by the review authors.

Synthesis

We categorized outcomes reported in these reviews into one of several domains (cognitive, clinical psychological, functional, physical, social, occupational, neurodegenerative diseases, and other outcomes). Within each domain, we grouped studies reporting similar outcomes and made qualitative judgments about the strength of the evidence for each outcome.

Included Systematic Reviews

Our initial combined search yielded 892 articles. An additional five citations came from searching other resources. We then conducted one round of abstract review and one round of full-text review and abstraction. Two reviewers shared the task of reviewing all 897 abstracts and the full-text versions of the 216 articles that passed the first screen. Seventy-two systematic reviews were included in our study. See Figure 2.1.

Characteristics of the Systematic Reviews

Systematic reviews included studies of a variety of adult populations. Approximately three-fourths of reviews included studies of the general adult population, about one-third of reviews

FIGURE 2.1

Flow Diagram of Included and Excluded Systematic Reviews Reporting the Risk or Prevalence of Long-Term Outcomes Following Traumatic Brain Injury

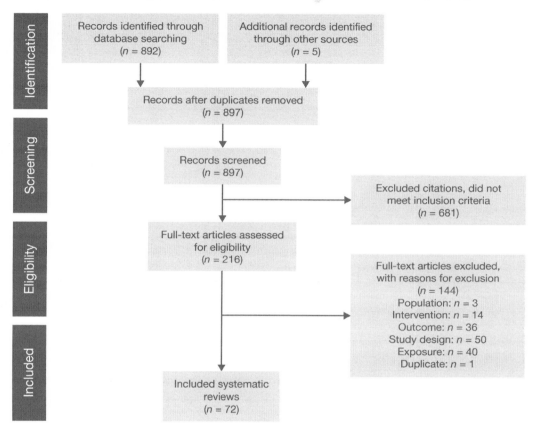

included studies of military or veteran populations, and about one-fourth included studies of athletes (usually professional or collegiate athletes). Studies also presented outcomes for a variety of time periods post-injury. We aimed to limit our focus to at least one year post-injury, but most reviews included studies with follow-up lengths that varied between six months and five to ten years post-injury. One review included studies that followed patients up to 70 years post-injury (Ozolins et al., 2016). A few reviews limited the post-injury time for study eligibility, but this was rarely a key facet of the systematic review or analysis. Many reviews did not report the average or range of time that patients were assessed post-injury and instead reported follow-up times for each individual included in the study.

About half of the reviews included TBI of all severity levels (mild, moderate, and severe). Some studies focused only on mild TBI or concussion or only on severe TBI. In our analysis, we separate the findings by TBI severity whenever possible. Studies varied in how they defined TBI severity; some used scales, such as the Glasgow Coma Scale, while others (often studies involving self-report of TBI) defined TBI severity according to whether a patient lost consciousness as a result of the TBI.

Reviews included searches of between one and ten databases, with an average (both mean and median) of four databases. Many reviews also included searches of reference lists of key articles, as well as searches through gray literature or the addition of articles based on knowledge of the authors. The systematic reviews included in our review were based on relatively recent searches of these databases. More than half of the reviews conducted their last searches for articles in 2015 or more recently, and more than 80 percent of the reviews conducted their last searches in 2011 or more recently.

Findings

TBI can have a widespread effect on long-term outcomes depending on the part of the brain that was injured and the circumstances surrounding the injury (e.g., whether there were other physical injuries). TBI is also associated with a variety of co-occurring conditions. In this section, we organize the findings on TBI outcomes into five domains: cognitive, functional, physical, social, and occupational. We organize the findings regarding co-occurring conditions into two categories: (1) psychological health conditions and health behaviors and (2) neurodegenerative conditions and other health conditions. As noted earlier, systematic reviews often did not report results by TBI severity.

Cognitive Outcomes

Cognitive outcomes included those related to attention, memory, and neurocognitive and executive function. On the whole, the literature suggests that long-term outcomes were worse for TBI patients across cognitive domains, such as memory and attention, although the strength of evidence varied depending on the cognitive domain, the severity of the TBI, and the time since the injury. Most studies of cognitive outcomes involved populations of athletes or the general population; only three focused on long-term cognitive outcomes among veterans, making it difficult to draw firm conclusions about the veteran population.

Attention and Memory

Seven systematic reviews indicated that long-term outcomes regarding attention and memory were worse for TBI patients than for others, although the findings were somewhat mixed depending on the population and how long it had been since the TBI. One review found that attention was worse in athletes with TBI than in those without (Zhang et al., 2019), while another review found no difference in attention outcomes (Cunningham et al., 2020). Several reviews found moderately poorer memory in athletes and other adults with TBI than without (Cunningham et al., 2020; Dunning, Westgate, and Adlam, 2016; Vakil et al., 2019; Zhang et al., 2019), and one review found that executive function was worse in those with TBI (Cunningham et al., 2020).

Four reviews suggested that changes in attention and cognition tended to resolve over time but did not resolve completely for those with more-severe TBI. One review found that most deficits in attention or cognition resolved within two years after TBI (Schultz and Tate, 2013), and a meta-analysis found that cognitive deficits resolved within three months for people with mild TBI (Belanger et al., 2005). Two other reviews indicated a similar improvement in outcomes over two years after moderate to severe TBI but also noted that some deficits remained after two years (Ruttan et al., 2008; Schretlen and Shapiro, 2003).

Overall Cognitive Function

Five reviews of cognitive function have focused on athletes, and some of this research has found an association between TBI and worse long-term cognitive function, although the strength of the evidence was relatively weak. One review found poorer cognitive function among athletes in rugby, American football, and boxing but noted that this result may not be clinically relevant (Gallo et al., 2020). One review found more self-reported cognitive difficulties among athletes with sport-related concussions compared with non-athletes and athletes in non-contact sports (Cunningham et al., 2020), and another found some studies suggesting higher prevalence of cognitive impairment in National Football League athletes (Schaffert et al., 2020). Another review of British soccer players with TBI also noted weak evidence for a relationship between TBI and neurocognitive impairment (Tarnutzer et al., 2017).

Among the general, and especially the veteran, population, results were more mixed and depended on the severity of TBI. Of the three reviews focusing on long-term cognitive outcomes among veteran populations, one review of outcomes in veterans and military personnel with mild TBI noted that few of the included studies identified an association with cognitive deficits (O'Neil et al., 2013). A review focusing on the general population found that reductions in cognitive function in patients with TBI were not significantly different from those in the rest of the population (Cunningham, Broglio, and Wilson, 2018). A review from 2009 found evidence of an association between more-severe TBI and neurocognitive deficits but insufficient evidence of an association between mild TBI and these deficits (Dikmen et al., 2009).

Functional Outcomes

There were relatively few articles looking at long-term functional outcomes after TBI, and we found none that looked at the effects of TBI on most activities of daily living. We identified only two reviews that looked at functional outcomes after TBI, including effects on the function of the motor system and the ability to drive a motor vehicle. One review found that repeated mild TBI was associated with a negative effect on the motor system, although the authors were not able to produce a pooled estimate because of the heterogeneity in the outcomes assessed (Ozolins et al., 2016). A review of the effects of TBI on driving found no increased risk of motor vehicle crash among people with TBI (Chee et al., 2019).

Physical Outcomes

Evidence from systematic reviews suggests that people with TBI have poorer physical long-term outcomes, including the prevalence of pain. We identified several reviews that assessed the prevalence or risk of certain physical outcomes after TBI, including physical or physiological symptoms, sleep, headache, and hearing. A review of the risk of musculoskeletal injury in athletes with TBI found increased odds of injury up to 24 months after injury (odds ratio [OR] = 2.11), with a higher point estimate for women (OR = 2.23) than men (OR = 2.06) (McPherson et al., 2019). Two reviews looked at pain in patients with TBI. One found that headache was present in one-third to one-half of patients five years after injury (Dobscha et al., 2009), with greater likelihood of headache in patients with co-occurring depression, PTSD, or insomnia. Another review found headache in 57.8 percent of patients and chronic pain in 51.5 percent of patients (Nampiaparampil, 2008). One review noted fatigue in patients with TBI but did not produce a point estimate of overall risk (Mollayeva et al., 2014). Despite the evidence provided in these reviews, given that people predisposed to TBI may already be at higher risk for these physical problems (e.g., musculoskeletal injuries), more evidence about the causal relationship between TBI and these outcomes is needed.

One review found that people with TBI had poorer sleep quality and shorter sleep duration (Grima et al., 2016), and another review found relatively high prevalence of visual deficits and dysfunctions in patients with TBI, including especially higher prevalence in those with moderate to severe TBI compared with those with mild TBI (Merezhinskaya et al., 2019). One review found overall low quality of evidence linking TBI and auditory dysfunction (Šarkić, Douglas, and Simpson, 2019). A review of adults with TBI found increased risk of stroke after TBI (hazard ratio = 1.86) but noted that the studies included in the review had heterogenous study designs and were low quality (Turner et al., 2021).

Social Outcomes

We identified only one review that looked at health-related quality of life. Polinder et al. (2015) found decreased quality of life using standard tools, such as the SF-36 short-form survey instrument, at least a year after TBI; the lowest scores were on the physical and emotional domains.

Occupational Outcomes

Two reviews explored occupational outcomes, including employment and return-to-work (reviews looking at return-to-work in the acute phase were excluded from our umbrella review because we were interested in long-term outcomes). The largest review of post-injury employment in the general population of patients with TBI (Gormley et al., 2019) found an overall employment rate of 42.2 percent, with an increase in the rate over time (35.0 percent at one-year post-injury, 42.1 percent up to five years post-injury, and 49.9 percent at five years and beyond). A smaller review (Cancelliere et al., 2014) found little evidence of the impact of TBI on returning to work.

Co-Occurring Psychological Health Conditions and Health Behaviors

TBI frequently co-occurs with other physical and psychological health conditions and can be associated with changes in certain health behaviors, such as substance use and suicidal thoughts, or with death by suicide. Co-occurring psychological health conditions constitute one of the most frequently studied domains; systematic reviews focused on such conditions as PTSD, depression, and anxiety. Several systematic reviews examined the relationship between TBI and health behaviors, such as substance misuse, aggression, violence, and suicide.

On the whole, the reviews suggest that TBI is associated with higher risk of a variety of psychological health conditions, although the strength of that relationship varies according to the condition studied. In addition, many reviews noted potential bias, including recall bias, in the diagnosis of these conditions and the relatively low prevalence of these psychological conditions overall.

PTSD

Four reviews addressed the risk of PTSD after TBI and found a strong and consistent association, although many reviews noted that they were unable to establish a causal relationship, given that there may be other underlying or confounding factors associated with both TBI and these psychological conditions. A review of veterans and civilians found prevalence of PTSD to be 27 percent in the TBI group and 11 percent in the non-TBI group, as well as a higher prevalence of PTSD in veterans with TBI (37 percent) than civilians with TBI (16 percent) (Loignon, Ouellet, and Belleville, 2020). Another review also found increased risk of PTSD in the military population with TBI (risk ratio = 2.33 after 12 months) compared with the civilian population with TBI (risk ratio = 1.70 after 12 months) (Iljazi et al., 2020). One review of PTSD did not separate by population and found an overall odds ratio of 1.73 among people with TBI and a pooled prevalence of PTSD of 15.6 percent (Van Praag et al., 2019). A fourth review found increased risk of PTSD but did not produce a point estimate (Greer et al., 2020).

Depression

Systematic reviews found a strong and consistent relationship between TBI and depression. Two reviews produced pooled estimates of depression risk after TBI. One found increased risk of depression (OR = 2.14) at least one year after injury, although the authors noted variability in study quality (Perry et al., 2016), while the other review found increased risk of depression after TBI, including an odds ratio of 3.42 at ten years after injury (Hellewell et al., 2020). Two reviews produced estimates of depression prevalence. One review found that the prevalence of depressive disorders in TBI patients at least one year after injury was 43 percent, with higher rates in women (Scholten et al., 2016), while another found depression in 24.5 percent of TBI patients (Rogers and Read, 2007). Two reviews of depression did not produce point estimates because of the heterogeneity of the included studies (Hutchison et al., 2018; Oyesanya and Ward, 2016), while others reported a qualitatively increased risk of depression without quantifying the risk (Greer et al., 2019; Hesdorffer, Rauch, and Tamminga, 2009; Manley et al., 2017; Vos, Nieuwenhuijsen, and Sluiter, 2018).

Anxiety

We identified only two reviews exploring the relationship between anxiety and TBI. Of these reviews, one found that the pooled prevalence of anxiety disorders one year after injury was slightly higher after a TBI (21 percent) than before the TBI (19 percent), with higher rates of anxiety after TBI in women (Scholten et al., 2016). The other review found increased risk of anxiety disorders after TBI but did not produce a point estimate (Greer et al., 2020).

Bipolar Disorder and Schizophrenia

Three reviews found increased risk of serious mental illness (bipolar disorder and schizophrenia) after TBI and produced point estimates of the increased risk. A review of bipolar disorder after TBI found increased risk (OR = 1.85) (Perry et al., 2016), as did a review of schizophrenia (OR = 1.65) (Molloy et al., 2011). Another review found schizophrenia in 4 percent of patients with TBI (Rogers and Read, 2007) compared with a prevalence of between 0.25 percent and 0.64 percent in the general population (National Institute of Mental Health, undated-b), although the authors noted that the included studies were inconsistent in terms of methods and findings. Review authors also noted that there is uncertainty about the potential biologic causal pathway between TBI and serious mental illness, and some reviews were unable to report on potential confounding factors, such as epilepsy.

Panic Disorder and Obsessive-Compulsive Disorder

One review found increased rates of other psychological outcomes, including panic disorder and obsessive-compulsive disorder. The review of psychiatric outcomes (Rogers and Read, 2007) found panic disorder in 4 percent of TBI patients (compared with 2.7-percent prevalence in the general population) and obsessive-compulsive disorder in 9.2 percent of TBI patients (compared with 1.2-percent prevalence in general population) (comparison numbers are from National Institute of Mental Health, undated-a).

Substance Use

The observed relationship between TBI and substance use differed across three reviews but leaned toward *decreased* rates of substance use after TBI. One review focused on substance abuse in general and found a decrease in substance use after moderate to severe TBI, no decrease after mild TBI, and a larger decrease after moderate to severe TBI in samples with more men than women (VanderVeen, 2021). However, another review that focused on veterans and military personnel reported increased risk of substance use disorder after TBI (Greer et al., 2020), although the authors noted that there was low strength of evidence for this increased risk. Finally, one review reported a pooled substance abuse prevalence of 11.5 percent in patients with TBI; however, this review did not control for demographic factors, and the authors noted that, given that substance use is a predictor of TBI, any observed high rates in substance use after TBI likely predate the injury (Rogers and Read, 2007).

Aggression and Violence

Three reviews explored the relationship between TBI and aggression or violence and generally found an increase in aggression after TBI. One produced a pooled odds ratio of violent behavior of 1.66 (Fazel et al., 2009), and another indicated increased risk of aggression in all included studies but noted that there was very little longitudinal follow-up in those studies (Buckley et al., 2017). A review from 2009 concluded that there was an association between TBI and aggressive behavior (Hesdorffer, Rauch, and Tamminga, 2009).

Suicide

Seven reviews explored the risk of suicide or suicidal ideation among TBI patients, with mixed results. One review found increased odds of suicide (risk ratio = 2.03) (Fralick et al., 2019). Another review found an elevated risk of suicide for people with severe TBI compared with those with mild TBI (hazard ratio = 1.4) (Simpson and Tate, 2007). One review found no increased risk of death by suicide among athletes (Manley et al., 2017), and three reviews did not produce point estimates of the risk of suicide (Bahraini et al., 2013; Greer et al., 2019; Greer et al., 2020). One review from 2009 found limited evidence of a link between TBI and death by suicide (Hesdorffer, Rauch, and Tamminga, 2009). Additionally, several reviews noted the potential for confounding with other conditions, including the underlying cause of the TBI.

Co-Occurring Neurodegenerative Disorders and Other Health Conditions

Several reviews explored the potential relationship between TBI and the subsequent development of other health conditions, including several neurodegenerative conditions. Overall, these reviews found mixed evidence for the relationship between TBI and dementia. Reviews found limited evidence for associations between TBI and other neurodegenerative conditions, such as amyotrophic lateral sclerosis (ALS) and Parkinson's disease, and conditions involving pituitary problems. However, these studies reported on relatively rare conditions and may have been limited by recall bias and other problems.

Dementia

Dementia was commonly studied as a potential outcome after TBI, although the findings were mixed and often varied by gender. We identified 12 reviews exploring the relationship between dementia (including Alzheimer's disease) and TBI. The earliest of these reviews, published in 2003, found a significantly greater risk of Alzheimer's disease overall (OR = 1.58) but found increased risk in men compared with women with TBI (OR = 2.26 and 0.92, respectively) (Fleminger et al., 2003). Another review, published in 2009, performed a qualitative synthesis, finding evidence of a link between moderate or severe TBI and subsequent development of Alzheimer's disease but insufficient evidence to link mild TBI with Alzheimer's disease (Bazarian et al., 2009). More-recent reviews have found pooled odds ratios for the risk of Alzheimer's disease or dementia to range between 1.03 and 1.96 (Huang et al., 2018; Li et al., 2017; Perry et al., 2016; Snowden et al., 2020), indicating a slightly higher risk relative to those without TBI (Li et al., 2017). Overall prevalence of dementia was reported in two reviews and ranged from 2.4 percent to 16 percent in populations with TBI and between 1.0 percent and 10 percent in similar populations without TBI (Huang et al., 2018; Peterson et al., 2020). Other reviews found no evidence linking mild TBI and development of dementia (Godbolt et al., 2014) or were limited by the poor quality of available studies or the heterogeneity of methods used (Gallo et al., 2020; Julien et al., 2017; Manley et al., 2017; Schaffert et al., 2020).

Amyotrophic Lateral Sclerosis

ALS was included as an outcome in five reviews. Two of these (Bazarian et al., 2009; Manley et al., 2017) were limited by low-quality studies with small sample sizes, but the three other reviews found that the pooled odds ratios of risk of ALS after TBI in the general population ranged between 1.38 and 2.97 (Huang et al., 2018; Liu et al., 2021; Watanabe and Watanabe, 2017). One of those reviews found an increased risk of ALS with more-severe injuries (OR = 1.69) (Liu et al., 2021). The other review found that ALS risk decreased with time, as the risk was not significantly greater than the baseline by three years after the injury (Watanabe and Watanabe, 2017).

Parkinson's Disease

The evidence for a relationship between TBI and Parkinson's disease was mixed and not as frequently studied as the relationship with dementia. Parkinson's disease was found to be associated with TBI in two reviews (Jafari et al., 2013; Perry et al., 2016), with odds ratios of 1.45 and 1.57, respectively. Another review found no association between Parkinson's and TBI (Huang et al., 2018). Three reviews were limited by a lack of high-quality studies or relatively few studies overall and did not provide point estimates of Parkinson's disease risk (Bazarian et al., 2009; Manley et al., 2017; Marras et al., 2014).

Pituitary Problems, Multiple Sclerosis, and Neoplasms

Other reviews found that TBI was associated with moderate increases in risk for certain other conditions. Three reviews looked at TBI patients' pituitary problems, which are quite rare in the general population. One of these reviews found that 31.6 percent of patients had an anterior pituitary disorder (e.g., hypopituitarism, growth hormone deficit, secondary adrenal failure) (Lauzier et al., 2014), while another found that 34 percent of patients in high-quality studies had one of these disorders (Emelifeonwu et al., 2020). One review found a high prevalence of hypopituitarism (27.5 percent) in patients with TBI, which was greater in patients with severe TBI than in those with mild or moderate TBI (Schneider et al., 2007). Another review found a small increase in the risk of multiple sclerosis (OR = 1.41), but this risk became statistically insignificant once low-quality studies were removed from the analysis (Warren et al., 2013). Another review found no evidence of increased risk of intracranial neoplasms (Rutherford and Wlodarczyk, 2009).

Additional Findings

In addition to the categories of outcomes and co-occurring conditions reported elsewhere in this section, we also noted several studies reporting on other outcomes. One review found generally poorer outcomes for patients with TBI in nursing homes, including increased risk of physically and verbally abusive behaviors (Kohnen et al., 2018). Another review found an unclear relationship between TBI and future criminal behavior (O'Sullivan et al., 2015). Another review of outcomes for veterans with TBI noted that, although rates of poor psychiatric outcomes were high in patients with TBI, there were few significant differences in outcomes between veterans with TBI and veterans without TBI (O'Neil et al., 2013). Other studies performed qualitative syntheses of a variety of outcomes in patients with TBI (Beadle et al., 2016; Carroll et al., 2014; Dikmen et al., 2009; Egeto et al., 2019; Mast et al., 2013; O'Neil et al., 2014).

Limitations of the Systematic Reviews

We noted many limitations (e.g., small sample sizes, recall bias) of both the systematic reviews included in our umbrella review and of the studies included in each of the reviews. All of the listed limitations discussed in this section were reported as a limitation by at least one review included in our umbrella review.

Limitations of Review Methodologies

Many of the included reviews had a heterogenous collection of outcomes (especially for such outcomes as cognitive function or clinical psychological outcomes, where included studies used a variety of scales or measures). When a pooled estimate of risk was produced (as was often the case with neurodegenerative disorders), often the review authors did not account for differences in control variables used in the individual included articles. About half of the reviews were limited by heterogeneity in assessing and reporting outcomes (especially those involving cognitive, social, or functional outcomes) and did not produce pooled estimates of risk or prevalence of outcomes. Most of these reviews presented qualitative syntheses of study results, often including an overall trend (i.e., "we find evidence of an association"), while others reported that there was not enough evidence to draw a conclusion. Some reviews included qualitative studies, which could not be aggregated into a pooled estimate of prevalence or risks of specific outcomes.

The reviews were also inconsistent in their review methodologies. Some used two reviewers for screening and abstraction and calculated concordance between reviewers (using Cohen's kappa), while others had only a single reviewer. Several reviews did not report key information, such as the dates when searches were run or the specific databases searched. Reviews were also inconsistent in which languages they allowed for included studies. All reviews included English-language articles, but some reviews allowed for other European or Asian languages.

Limitations of Included Studies

One of the most commonly cited limitations by authors of the reviews was potential selection bias in the population covered in the included studies (e.g., convenience samples of athletes, samples of those seeking treatment at medical facilities). Some studies also had small sample sizes (less than 100 participants). Included case-control studies were often limited by recall bias or self-reported data, for both the number and severity of TBIs incurred. Studies also used differing definitions of TBI and differing scales to assess TBI. Most studies included a range of TBI severity, but others focused on a single severity categorization (e.g., mild TBI). Some studies used clinical diagnosis of TBI, but others relied on self-report. For many reviews, especially those not specifically focused on a clinical condition as an outcome, included studies used differing definitions of various outcomes (e.g., criminal behavior).

Reviews often noted a general low quality of evidence in included studies, usually based on standardized assessments of study quality. These low-quality assessments were often driven by missing information. Studies also controlled for different sets of potential confounders, which limited the generalizability of some findings (i.e., if one study included in a review controlled for a variety of factors but other studies did not control for those factors). Publication bias was sometimes listed as a limitation, but other studies used funnel plots and Egger's tests to systematically assess the risk of publication bias.

Summary

We found a large number of systematic reviews and meta-analyses that explored the relationship between TBI and long-term outcomes. The ability to measure changes in long-term outcomes was limited. Systematic reviews examined long-term outcomes after TBI across several domains, including cognitive outcomes, such as memory and attention; physical outcomes, such as headaches and sleep quality; and co-occurring health conditions, such as PTSD, depression, dementia, ALS, and Parkinson's disease.

Of all outcome domains, the most commonly studied were co-occurring psychological conditions and subsequently developed health conditions. Many reviews found increased odds or risk of these negative outcomes. Relatively few reviews reported prevalence of these long-term outcomes, and those that did showed an increased pooled odds ratio or relative risk often estimated as a small overall absolute risk increase in the long term. Several studies that stratified outcomes by the number of years post-injury even found decreasing odds of negative outcomes with time.

Very few reviews looked at functional, social, or occupational outcomes, which are often important outcomes for patients. We did not identify any reviews that produced a quantitative assessment of the impact of TBI on health care costs. Reviews that incorporated weights by evidence quality or that limited analyses to medium- or high-quality evidence found a smaller effect of TBI on negative outcomes; we noted when reporting results if a review incorporated evidence quality. Many studies noted that they were not able to establish causation, especially for PTSD, which may be caused by an unobserved confounding variable that also caused the TBI (e.g., blast trauma), a layer of complexity that is highly relevant to the post-9/11 veteran population. Very few of the reviews included only veteran populations; given the unique experiences and needs of this population, the applicability of reviews of TBI in athletes or the general adult population may be limited.

Additionally, very few reviews (less than 20 percent) accounted for gender when assessing TBI outcomes. In the few reviews that did include gender as a dimension of analysis, differential outcomes by gender were often observed, indicating that future research into TBI outcomes should take gender into account. Even fewer reviews looked at outcomes by race or ethnicity, suggesting an important area for future research.

Many reviews were also relatively inconsistent in the length of follow-up of included studies. The follow-up in these included studies often ranged from one to ten or more years. About half of the reviews included TBI of all severity levels (mild, moderate, and severe), while some studies focused only on mild TBI or concussion or only on severe TBI. Several reviews identified a period of improvement in outcomes up to two years after injury, so future reviews and studies should be mindful of the potential differences in outcomes by time after TBI.

CHAPTER THREE

Characteristics of WWP Alumni with Traumatic Brain Injury and Other Head Injuries

WWP invests significant resources to learn more about the population it serves by conducting the Annual Warrior Survey of its alumni. These survey responses are used to inform WWP's advocacy efforts. They also provide a data-driven approach to ensure that WWP is serving the populations that it intends to serve, learn about what additional services it can provide to meet those populations' needs, and identify how subpopulations differ from one another so that WWP can learn whether there are unique needs or gaps that need to be addressed.

The last of these goals is the key objective of this chapter. We used three years (2017, 2018, 2020) of survey data, which we received from WWP, to understand how veterans who self-reported experiencing a head injury differed from those who did not.[1] Respondents were identified as having a head injury if they reported either (1) TBI or (2) head injuries other than TBI.[2] The focus of this report is on TBI, but because of a concern that TBI is underreported, we chose to examine the broader population of individuals with a head injury. There may be biases in self-reports of either TBI or other head injuries (for example, some groups of veterans may be less likely to self-report having conditions), and the survey does not collect information about severity of injury or specific symptoms experienced by respondents.

It is important to note that the WWP alumni population does not represent the full population of veterans. WWP alumni are a unique subset of the U.S. veteran population. First, the population includes only a subset of those who may experience physical and mental health problems. The eligibility criteria to become a WWP alumnus indicate that such problems

---

[1] We use the term *veterans* when describing WWP survey results but acknowledge that some alumni are still serving in the military (see Table 3.3 later in this chapter).

[2] Survey respondents were asked to "choose all that apply" to indicate "any severe physical or mental injuries or health problems you experienced while serving, or as a result of serving, in the military after September 11, 2001." Response options included "traumatic brain injury (TBI)" and "head injuries other than traumatic brain injury (TBI)."

must have developed while or be in relation to serving in the military. Many other veterans may experience physical and mental health problems unrelated to their military service. Second, the WWP alumni population served in the military after 9/11, which makes them younger, on average, than other veteran groups (e.g., Vietnam-era veterans). Third, joining WWP requires that an individual register and submit documentation of military service and indicate a physical or mental health–related concern. Thus, this is a help-seeking group of veterans (or their family members), and their level of need may be higher than others who did not choose to join WWP. Given these distinctions, care should be taken when interpreting how the findings related to the WWP alumni presented in this report generalize to other veterans who served pre-9/11 and other post-9/11 veterans who have not sought assistance from WWP.

Approach to the Analysis of WWP Survey Data

We analyzed aggregated data from the 2017, 2018, and 2020 cross-sectional Annual Warrior Surveys (response rates across survey years are provided in Appendix B).[3] Although these cross-sectional surveys differ slightly year to year, they provide a largely overlapping set of items, allowing us to leverage all these data jointly. Our approach also means that there may be overlap in respondents across years; however, because of the anonymous format of the data, we were unable to characterize respondent overlap across years. Across all three years, we identified a sample of 43,150 respondents with a head injury and 53,021 without a head injury. Differences across years are presented in Table 3.1. For all analyses, we used the post-stratification weights developed by the survey vendor.

Because we conducted several statistical tests, we expected to detect many false positive findings using conventional ($p < 0.05$) thresholds. Additionally, because of our large sample size, we expected to find many highly significant results with small effect sizes. We also were aware that there may be non-independence of observations, particularly for veterans who responded to the survey in more than one year. To address each of these issues, we identified differences that meet two criteria: (1) A statistical test between the two groups meets a

TABLE 3.1
WWP Survey Sample Size, by Survey Year and Head Injury Status

Survey Year	With a Head Injury	Without a Head Injury
2017	15,989	18,833
2018	15,341	17,726
2020	11,820	16,462
All	43,150	53,021

---

[3] We did not include the 2019 survey because it was administered differently and in a way that did not permit easy aggregation with the 2017, 2018, and 2020 surveys.

very conservative p-value threshold ($p < 0.0001$),[4] and (2) the difference is at least 2 percentage points. Across tables in this chapter, we highlight these differences with an asterisk in the p-value column, and we typically describe them in the text. For each level of a categorical variable, we highlight differences of at least 2 percentage points when the chi-square test (incorporating all levels of the variable) meets our p-value threshold. In the tables, we identify the p-value in the top, shaded row for chi-square analyses. We identify the p-value in each row for pairwise comparisons.

Results

Demographic Characteristics

Most of the tables in this chapter are similar in structure, so we closely guide readers through the results presented in Table 3.2, and we provide less explanation about the results in subsequent tables. First, there was evidence of gender differences between survey respondents with and without a head injury. Specifically, women constituted 11 percent of those with a head injury, compared with 23 percent of those without a head injury. There were also age differences between the groups. The population of veterans with a head injury included more individuals 31 to 45 years old (64 percent) relative to the population of veterans without a head injury (59 percent). The population with a head injury also had fewer individuals 46 to 60 years old than did the population without a head injury (24 percent versus 26 percent, respectively). And there were differences worth noting across all education groups: More of those in the head injury group had less than a high school degree (12 percent versus 9 percent) and had completed some college, business, or vocational education (40 percent versus 34 percent). Conversely, fewer veterans in the head injury group had obtained an associate's or bachelor's degree (38 percent versus 41 percent) or completed more than a college degree (11 percent versus 16 percent).

There were interesting differences by race and ethnicity. For instance, 61 percent of those with a head injury identified as white, non-Hispanic relative to 54 percent of those without a head injury, and 6 percent of those with a head injury identified as American Indian or Alaska Native relative to 4 percent of those without a head injury. Conversely, 9 percent of those with a head injury identified as Black, non-Hispanic relative to 17 percent of those without a head injury. Finally, 68 percent of the respondents with a head injury were married, compared with 64 percent of those without a head injury, and 9 percent of the head injury respondents were single, compared with 13 percent of the group without a head injury. We observed no differences meeting our 2-percentage-point group difference by housing status, although there were statistically significant differences below that threshold between the two groups.

---

[4] We chose the $p < 0.0001$ threshold because it is approximately equivalent to the Bonferroni correction, controlling the family-wise error rate at 0.05.

TABLE 3.2

Demographic Characteristics of WWP Survey Respondents, by Head Injury Status

Characteristic	With Head Injury (%)	Without Head Injury (%)	p-Value
Gender			< 0.0001
Men	89.23	77.14	*
Women	10.77	22.86	*
Age			< 0.0001
18–30	10.43	12.02	
31–45	64.35	59.21	*
46–60	23.57	26.05	*
61+	1.66	2.73	
Educational attainment			< 0.0001
< High school diploma, high school diploma, or GED diploma	11.5	9.42	*
Some college, business, or vocational education	39.52	33.52	*
Associate's or bachelor's degree	37.51	41.44	*
More than a college degree	11.46	15.62	*
Race/ethnicity			< 0.0001
White, non-Hispanic	61.05	54.22	*
Black, non-Hispanic	9.18	16.65	*
Hispanic	16.64	18.16	
American Indian or Alaska Native	6.03	3.80	*
Asian	3.02	3.61	
Native Hawaiian	1.76	1.44	
Other	2.31	2.11	
Marital status			< 0.0001
Married	68.44	64.56	*
Widowed	0.48	0.50	
Divorced	17.92	18.41	
Separated	4.22	3.78	
Single	8.93	12.75	*

Table 3.2—Continued

Characteristic	With Head Injury (%)	Without Head Injury (%)	p-Value
Housing status			< 0.0001
Live in military housing	1.75	2.08	
Rent or own my own home	87.94	87.13	
Share a dwelling	8.24	8.67	
Live alone	0.32	0.32	
Transitional or Section 8 housing	0.84	1.10	
Supported housing, assisted-living facility, or nursing home	0.38	0.33	
Homeless or living in a shelter	0.54	0.37	

NOTE: GED = Tests of General Educational Development.

* An asterisk indicates that p < 0.0001, and the difference between the two groups was at least 2 percentage points.

Military Characteristics

There were significant differences across most military characteristics we examined (Table 3.3). Fewer of those in the head injury group were currently serving in the reserves or National Guard (4 percent) than those in the group without a head injury (7 percent). A greater share of those with head injury who were no longer serving had been medically retired or were discharged or separated, and a smaller share had been non-medically retired, compared with the shares of those without a head injury who were no longer serving—a logical difference between the groups. More veterans with a head injury had served in the Army and Marine Corps, and fewer had served in the Navy, Air Force, or a category consisting of Coast Guard, National Guard, and reserve service members (which we combined because of how the question was asked in one or more survey years). Although there were no major differences between groups in the percentage of officers or warrant officers, there were among the enlisted service members. The head injury group had fewer junior enlisted (57 percent versus 59 percent) and more senior enlisted (36 percent versus 32 percent). Finally, the head injury group had a greater share of those with between two and four deployments (50 percent versus 45 percent) and five or more deployments (25 percent versus 21 percent), while the group without a head injury had a greater share of those with less than two deployments.

TABLE 3.3

Military Characteristics of WWP Survey Respondents, by Head Injury Status

Characteristic	With Head Injury (%)	Without Head Injury (%)	p-Value
Current military service			
Current active duty	5.73	7.13	< 0.0001
Current reserves or National Guard	4.06	6.86	< 0.0001*
No longer serving			< 0.0001
Retired – medical	53.16	33.19	*
Retired – non-medical	11.85	18.06	*
Discharged or separated	35.00	48.75	*
Service branch[a]			< 0.0001
Army	71.18	60.50	*
Marine Corps	17.13	13.40	*
Air Force	6.93	13.09	*
Navy	8.74	13.85	*
Coast Guard, National Guard, or reserves	21.98	24.86	*
Highest rank			< 0.0001
E1–E5	56.90	59.11	*
E6–E9	35.70	31.85	*
Warrant officer	1.23	1.40	
Officer	6.17	7.65	
Deployments			< 0.0001
0	2.33	7.91	*
1	22.47	27.03	*
2–4	50.38	44.46	*
5 or more	24.82	20.59	*

* An asterisk indicates that $p < 0.0001$, and the difference between the two groups was at least 2 percentage points.

[a] For service branch, respondents who served in multiple branches over their careers are included in each relevant category.

Use of WWP Programs and Services

The Annual Warrior Survey asked about alumni's use of a variety of WWP services, listed in Table 3.4. The only difference we observed between the two groups that met our criteria was enrollment in Project Odyssey or the Combat Stress Recovery Program.[5] More of those with a head injury (7 percent) used this service, relative to the group without a head injury (4 percent).

TABLE 3.4

WWP Services Used by WWP Survey Respondents, by Head Injury Status

WWP Service or Program	With Head Injury (%)	Without Head Injury (%)	p-Value
Alumni events (e.g., those advertised in The Post)[a]	28.96	28.42	0.0574
Benefits counseling	10.33	10.38	0.4500
Emergency financial assistance	5.82	5.69	0.1992
Collegiate sports events with WWP	4.44	3.62	0.0009
Independence Program	3.08	1.36	< 0.0001
Peer support groups	7.96	6.46	< 0.0001
Physical health and wellness events or coaching	11.94	11.02	< 0.0001
WWP adaptive sports events	4.43	3.09	< 0.0001
Policy, legislation, or advocacy	1.76	1.41	< 0.0001
Project Odyssey or the Combat Stress Recovery Program	6.66	4.37	< 0.0001*
Warrior Care Network	4.15	2.98	< 0.0001
WWP Resource Center	10.11	9.04	< 0.0001
Soldier Ride	4.72	3.84	< 0.0001
Warriors to Work	6.49	7.50	< 0.0001
WWP Backpacks	1.58	1.22	< 0.0001
WWP Talk	3.25	2.84	< 0.0001
Other activities and events	15.11	13.74	< 0.0001
I do not know	3.94	3.55	< 0.0001
I have not participated in programs through WWP in the past 12 months	38.38	39.71	< 0.0001

* An asterisk indicates that $p < 0.0001$, and the difference between the two groups was at least 2 percentage points.

[a] The Post is a weekly email highlighting upcoming WWP events.

---

[5] Project Odyssey is a 12-week adventure-based learning mental health program; the Combat Stress Recovery Program addresses the mental health and cognitive needs of veterans at key stages during readjustment.

Utilization and Receipt of VA and Other Health Benefits

Survey respondents with a head injury and those without indicated differences in their utilization and receipt of VA and other health benefits (Table 3.5). Most notably, a greater share of those with a head injury than those without a head injury received VA compensation benefits (95 percent versus 91 percent) and relied on VA as their primary care provider (74 percent versus 68 percent). There was also a trend with respect to military Physical Evaluation Board disability ratings: Compared with shares of respondents without a head injury, smaller shares of those with a head injury had no disability rating or a rating of less than 30 percent, but larger shares reported having disability ratings higher than 30 percent. With respect to VA service-connected disability ratings, 49 percent of those with a head injury and 27 percent of those without a head injury had a rating of 100 percent. Also, a greater percentage of those with a head injury were receiving health insurance through Medicare (which is the federal program for the elderly and disabled), VA, and TRICARE (the health care program for active-duty military members, their families, and military retirees), but a smaller percentage had employer- or union-sponsored health insurance (17 percent versus 26 percent).

TABLE 3.5

Utilization and Receipt of VA and Other Health Benefits Among WWP Survey Respondents, by Head Injury Status

Benefit	With Head Injury (%)	Without Head Injury (%)	p-Value
VA compensation			
Receiving VA compensation benefits[a]	94.57	91.00	< 0.0001*
VA service-connected disability rating			< 0.0001
No disability rating/has claim pending or on appeal	7.08	11.01	*
<30%	0.96	4.39	*
30–60%	9.22	20.88	*
70–90%	34.06	36.79	*
100%	48.68	26.93	*
Military Physical Evaluation Board disability rating			< 0.0001
No disability rating or claim pending or on appeal	46.63	61.16	*
<30%	4.96	6.46	
30–60%	17.67	15.49	*
70–90%	19.88	11.13	*
100%	10.87	5.75	*

Table 3.5—Continued

Benefit	With Head Injury (%)	Without Head Injury (%)	p-Value
Health insurance[b]			
None	2.24	2.59	0.0034
Current or former employer or union	17.15	25.91	< 0.0001*
Purchased directly from an insurance company	1.66	1.58	0.9645
Medicare	19.39	9.91	< 0.0001*
Medicaid or medical assistance	4.59	3.12	< 0.0001
VA	77.17	70.44	< 0.0001*
TRICARE	52.56	42.47	< 0.0001*
Care provision			
VA is primary care provider	73.94	67.80	< 0.0001*

* An asterisk indicates that $p < 0.0001$, and the difference between the two groups was at least 2 percentage points.

[a] Receiving VA compensation benefits excludes those with a VA claim pending or on appeal.

[b] Respondents were allowed to indicate more than one type of health insurance.

Utilization of Education Benefits

Earlier in this chapter, we noted that the percentage of WWP survey respondents with a head injury who had attained an associate's, bachelor's, or higher degree was smaller than the percentage of respondents without a head injury who had attained those degrees. Surprisingly, we saw no differences between groups in the percentage currently enrolled in school (22 percent in each group) (Table 3.6). However, among WWP respondents enrolled in school, a higher share of those with a head injury than those without were using VA or other government benefits to access schooling (85 percent versus 82 percent).

Employment and Employability

There were differences between the groups on most domains related to employment and employability (Table 3.7). Relative to those without a head injury, fewer of those with a head injury were currently employed full time, were looking for work, or worked 35 hours per week or more over the past year. In addition, fewer of those with a head injury were satisfied with work. Among respondents not currently working, a greater share of those with a head injury reported being unable to return to work because of a temporary illness, and a greater share reported not looking for work because of a physical or mental injury from a service-connected disability. The survey also asked about factors that would make it difficult to obtain employment or change jobs. Compared with the share of respondents without a head injury, a greater share of those with a head injury reported that each factor that was presented in the survey—loss of financial benefits, loss of medical benefits, not physically able,

TABLE 3.6

Utilization of Education Benefits Among WWP Survey Respondents, by Head Injury Status

Benefit	With Head Injury (%)	Without Head Injury (%)	p-Value
Currently enrolled in school	21.70	22.40	0.0481
Using any VA or government benefits to access schooling (conditional on being enrolled in school)	84.85	81.90	< 0.0001*

* An asterisk indicates that p < 0.0001, and the difference between the two groups was at least 2 percentage points.

TABLE 3.7

Employment and Employability Characteristics Among WWP Survey Respondents, by Head Injury Status

Characteristic	With Head Injury (%)	Without Head Injury (%)	p-Value
Employment status			
Currently employed – full time	38.56	52.79	< 0.0001*
Currently employed – part time	7.13	7.92	< 0.0001
Currently looking for work	20.28	26.24	< 0.0001*
Worked 35 hours per week or more each week in past 12 months	78.78	82.54	< 0.0001*
Work satisfaction (among those employed full or part time)			
Satisfied, very satisfied, or totally satisfied with work	49.57	53.28	< 0.0001*
Health condition affecting employment (among those not currently working)			
Could not return to work last week if recalled (or started a new job) because of a temporary illness	11.14	8.74	0.0006
Not looking for work because of a physical or mental injury from a service-connected disability	38.54	35.38	< 0.0001*
Indicated that the following factors would make it more difficult to obtain employment or change jobs			
Would lose financial benefits (e.g., disability)	12.37	6.73	< 0.0001*
Would lose medical benefits	6.70	4.27	< 0.0001*
Not physically capable	25.08	15.49	< 0.0001*
Mental health issues	40.28	26.59	< 0.0001*
Psychological distress or hopelessness	23.63	15.52	< 0.0001*
Difficult to be around others	35.40	22.01	< 0.0001*
Unable to get hired because of injury or disability	14.81	7.57	< 0.0001*

* An asterisk indicates that p < 0.0001, and the difference between the two groups was at least 2 percentage points.

mental health issues, psychological distress or hopelessness, difficulty being around others, and inability to get hired because of injury or disability—would make it difficult to find or switch jobs.

Other Physical or Mental Injuries

All WWP alumni were asked whether they had a series of other physical or mental injuries, such as hearing loss, military sexual trauma, and sleep problems (Table 3.8). For all but two physical and mental ailments, the share of those with a head injury who endorsed the ailment was greater than the share of those without a head injury who did so, and the difference met our predefined threshold for an asterisk. The two exceptions were that the difference between the share with an amputation was less than 2 percentage points, and a lower share of those with a head injury reported having experienced a military sexual trauma (8 percent versus 10 percent)—possibly a reflection of the gender differences between the groups, as described earlier.

TABLE 3.8
Other Physical and Mental Injuries Among WWP Survey Respondents, by Head Injury Status

Injury	With Head Injury (%)	Without Head Injury (%)	p-Value
Physical injury			
Amputation	2.12	1.05	< 0.0001
Ankle or feet injuries	39.84	32.66	< 0.0001*
Back, neck, or shoulder problems	80.11	68.20	< 0.0001*
Blind or severe visual loss	3.03	0.81	< 0.0001*
Burns (severe)	3.12	0.80	< 0.0001*
Fractured bones	21.44	10.91	< 0.0001*
Hand injuries	23.04	12.49	< 0.0001*
Hearing loss	62.22	37.59	< 0.0001*
Hip injuries	18.12	12.87	< 0.0001*
Knee injuries or problems	58.87	48.56	< 0.0001*
Migraines or other severe headaches	67.77	34.37	< 0.0001*
Military sexual trauma	7.87	10.05	< 0.0001*
Nerve injuries	36.08	20.46	< 0.0001*
Shrapnel problems	11.47	1.91	< 0.0001*
Spinal cord injury	18.17	8.55	< 0.0001*

Table 3.8—Continued

Injury	With Head Injury (%)	Without Head Injury (%)	p-Value
Tinnitus	71.06	50.13	< 0.0001*
Other severe physical injuries	16.05	12.16	< 0.0001*
Mental injury			
Anxiety	77.86	66.00	< 0.0001*
Depression	77.13	66.01	< 0.0001*
PTSD	90.93	70.36	< 0.0001*
Sleep problems	86.04	71.92	< 0.0001*
Other severe mental injuries	13.73	7.79	< 0.0001*

* An asterisk indicates that $p < 0.0001$, and the difference between the two groups was at least 2 percentage points.

Caregiver Support

The Annual Warrior Survey asked whether the veteran or service member requires caregiver support and, if so, about characteristics of that support. Almost one-third (29 percent) of the group with a head injury required caregiver support, and, of those respondents, 28 percent were enrolled in VA's Program of Comprehensive Assistance for Family Caregivers. Those numbers compare with 16 percent of those without a head injury who required caregiver support, and, of those respondents, 16 percent were enrolled in VA's Program of Comprehensive Assistance for Family Caregivers. Among those needing caregiver support, a greater share of those with a head injury reported that the caregiver was a spouse (85 percent versus 82 percent), whereas a smaller share of those with a head injury relied on other family besides a spouse or parent. And a greater percentage of those with a head injury were housebound (11 percent versus 6 percent).

Respondents also were asked about specific activities for which they required assistance. For every activity, the share of those with a head injury who indicated requiring assistance was greater than the share of those without a head injury who indicated that need (Table 3.9). The activities that veterans needed support with the most were taking medications properly (49 percent of the group with a head injury versus 24 percent of the group without a head injury), doing household chores (48 percent versus 31 percent), and managing money (45 percent versus 25 percent). The activities that veterans needed assistance with the least were toileting (11 percent versus 6 percent) and using the telephone (11 percent versus 5 percent).

The survey also asked about the time that caregivers spend performing caregiving duties. According to the survey results, caregivers to those with a head injury spent more time per week than caregivers to those without a head injury. Specifically, 18 percent of caregivers to veterans with a head injury spent 21–30 hours per week, 10 percent spent 31–40 hours per

TABLE 3.9

Caregiver Support Among WWP Survey Respondents, by Head Injury Status

Caregiver Support Characteristic	With Head Injury (%)	Without Head Injury (%)	p-Value
Require caregiver support because of any physical or mental injuries or health problems experienced while serving in the military after September 11, 2001	29.22	16.04	< 0.0001*
Among those receiving caregiver support			
Enrolled in the Program of Comprehensive Assistance for Family Caregivers	28.01	16.12	< 0.0001*
Veteran is housebound	11.22	5.53	< 0.0001*
Caregiver relationship to spouse			0.0039
Caregiver is spouse	85.27	81.93	
Caregiver is parent	7.02	6.47	
Caregiver is other family	3.23	5.34	
Caregiver is other person	4.48	6.26	
Veteran requires ANY assistance with . . .			
Taking medications properly	48.65	23.83	< 0.0001*
Doing household chores	47.89	30.55	< 0.0001*
Managing money	45.10	25.33	< 0.0001*
Preparing meals	33.82	17.53	< 0.0001*
Dressing and undressing	25.28	13.60	< 0.0001*
Bathing	23.55	12.02	< 0.0001*
Grooming	22.72	11.53	< 0.0001*
Mobility	19.86	10.53	< 0.0001*
Eating	13.17	5.72	< 0.0001*
Prosthetic adjustment or use of assistive devices	11.93	6.32	< 0.0001*
Toileting	11.47	5.60	< 0.0001*
Using the telephone	10.92	4.85	< 0.0001*

* An asterisk indicates that $p < 0.0001$, and the difference between the two groups was at least 2 percentage points.

week, and 26 percent spent more than 40 hours per week; in contrast, those numbers were 16 percent, 8 percent, and 19 percent, respectively, for caregivers to those without a head injury (Figure 3.1).

FIGURE 3.1

Time Spent Performing Caregiving Duties, by Head Injury Status

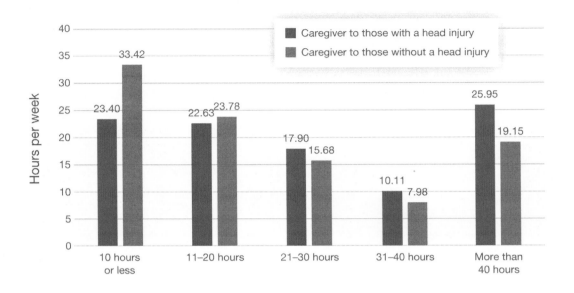

We employed regression analysis to test whether caring for someone with a head injury was independently associated with time spent performing caregiving duties and, separately, whether the caregiver's relationship with the warrior was independently associated with time spent caregiving. In these analyses, we examined only the bivariate relationship between each caregiving factor and time spent performing caregiving duties, without adjustment for other factors. We then employed multivariate regression to test whether caregiving for someone with a head injury was associated with time spent caregiving, after accounting for the caregiver's relationship to the warrior and other factors, including the total number of physical and mental injuries and the number of activities requiring assistance. In bivariate (unadjusted) models, caring for a veteran with a head injury was associated with time spent caregiving (Table 3.10), similar to what is shown in Figure 3.1. However, once we accounted for the caregiver's relationship to the warrior, the total number of physical and mental injuries, and the total number of activities for which a person required assistance, the relationship between head injury and time spent caregiving was no longer significant ($p = 0.09$). In other words, caregivers to those with a head injury spent more time performing caregiving duties likely because those veterans had a greater number of mental injuries and a greater number of activities requiring caregiver assistance. Table 3.10 reports the beta coefficient (β), representing the estimated change in the outcome associated with a given predictor, and the p-value for these unadjusted and adjusted analyses.

TABLE 3.10

Predictors of Time Spent Performing Caregiver Duties

Predictor	Bivariate (Unadjusted)		Adjusted	
	β	p-Value	β	p-Value
Veteran has head injury	0.27	< 0.0001	0.08	0.0615
Caregiver relationship to spouse				
Caregiver is spouse (reference)				
Caregiver is parent	−0.10	0.2063	−0.01	0.8946
Caregiver is other family	−0.46	< 0.0001	−0.43	< 0.0001
Caregiver is other person	−0.35	0.0002	−0.27	0.0029
Total number of physical injuries	0.06	< 0.0001	0.01	0.0645
Total number of mental injuries	0.16	< 0.0001	0.11	< 0.0001
Total number of activities requiring assistance	0.15	< 0.0001	0.14	< 0.0001

Self-Reported Health

Self-reported health is a single item in the Annual Warrior Survey that asked respondents to rate their overall health from poor to excellent. A greater share of those with a head injury than of those without a head injury reported their health as poor (13 percent versus 8 percent) or fair (44 percent versus 37 percent). Correspondingly, a smaller share reported their health as good (34 percent versus 39 percent) or very good (8 percent versus 13 percent). See Table 3.11.

We again used regression analysis to test whether those with a head injury reported worse overall health, controlling for the total number of physical and mental injuries, the total number of activities for which the veteran required assistance, and hazardous drinking and drug use (described further later in this chapter). We also adjusted for the total number of WWP programs that the veteran participated in and the veteran's demographic characteristics (age, gender, educational attainment, race/ethnicity, marital status, and housing status). We first examined the relationship between one factor and another independently (e.g., the relationship between head injury and self-reported health, without adjusting for any other variables) and then simultaneously (e.g., the relationship between head injury and self-reported health, adjusting for the variables just described). Interestingly, without adjustment, having a head injury was associated with lower self-reported health, but after accounting for these factors, having a head injury was associated with *higher* self-reported health (unadjusted $\beta = -0.24$, p < 0.01; adjusted $\beta = 0.04$, p < 0.01). Also, after adjustment, the total number of WWP programs that the veteran participated in was associated with higher self-reported health (Table 3.12; the full table with demographic characteristics is presented in Appendix B).

TABLE 3.11

Self-Reported Health Among WWP Survey Respondents, by Head Injury Status

Self-Reported Health	With Head Injury (%)	Without Head Injury (%)	p-Value
Poor	12.69	8.14	< 0.0001*
Fair	43.92	36.69	< 0.0001*
Good	33.67	39.30	< 0.0001*
Very good	8.21	13.15	< 0.0001*
Excellent	1.50	2.72	< 0.0001

* An asterisk indicates that $p < 0.0001$, and the difference between the two groups was at least 2 percentage points.

TABLE 3.12

Predictors of Self-Reported Health

Predictor	Bivariate (Unadjusted)		Adjusted	
	β	p-Value	β	p-Value
Veteran has head injury	−0.24	< 0.0001	0.04	< 0.0001
Total number of physical injuries	−0.09	< 0.0001	−0.04	< 0.0001
Total number of mental injuries	−0.21	< 0.0001	−0.13	< 0.0001
Total number of activities requiring assistance	−0.11	< 0.0001	−0.08	< 0.0001
Total number of WWP programs that the veteran participates in	−0.02	< 0.0001	0.02	< 0.0001
Hazardous drinking	0.03	< 0.0001	0.00	0.9417
Drug use	−0.17	< 0.0001	−0.03	< 0.0001

Mental Health Symptoms

Veterans who complete the survey are asked about mental health symptoms with scales that measure depression and PTSD. Specifically, depression was measured with the 9-item Patient Health Questionnaire, which asks about nine depressive symptoms in the past two weeks. The scale ranges from 0 to 27, and scores of ten or higher indicate probable depression (Kroenke, Spitzer, and Williams, 2001). PTSD symptoms were assessed with the PTSD Checklist for DSM-5, which consists of 20 questions that map onto criteria from the *Diagnostic and Statistical Manual of Mental Disorders*, 5th edition. Scores range from 0 to 80, and scores of 31 or greater are considered probable PTSD cases (Weathers et al., 2013).[6] Using

---

[6] PTSD symptoms were obtained from only the 2020 survey, when the PTSD Checklist for DSM-5 was administered.

these thresholds, a greater share of those with a head injury than those without a head injury met probable criteria for depression (68 percent versus 53 percent) and PTSD (67 percent versus 50 percent) (Table 3.13).

As we did with self-reported health, we used regression analysis to test whether those with a head injury had elevated depression and PTSD symptoms, controlling for the total number of physical and mental injuries, the total number of activities for which the veteran required assistance, and hazardous drinking and drug use. We also adjusted for the total number of WWP programs that the veteran participated in and the veteran's demographic characteristics (age, gender, educational attainment, race/ethnicity, marital status, and housing status). For both outcomes, head injury was independently associated with greater symptom severity (depression: adjusted $\beta = 0.12$, $p = 0.0039$; PTSD: adjusted $\beta = 1.44$, $p < 0.0001$) (Table 3.14).

Sleep Quality

The 2020 Annual Warrior Survey also included questions on sleep quality, using a scale called the Pittsburgh Sleep Quality Index (Buysse et al., 1989). The scale value ranges from 0 to 21, and higher scores indicate worse sleep quality. We again used regression analysis to test whether those with a head injury had poorer sleep quality, controlling for the total number of physical and mental injuries, the total number of activities for which the veteran required assistance, and hazardous drinking and drug use. We also adjusted for the total number of WWP programs that the veteran participated in and the veteran's demographic characteristics (age, gender, educational attainment, race/ethnicity, marital status, and housing status). Although having a head injury was associated with poorer sleep quality before accounting for other factors (unadjusted $\beta = 1.44$, $p < 0.0001$), after adjustment, the association was no longer significant (adjusted $\beta = 0.09$, $p = 0.0848$) (Table 3.15).

TABLE 3.13

Prevalence of Depression and PTSD Symptoms Among WWP Survey Respondents, by Head Injury Status

Mental Health Condition	With Head Injury (%)	Without Head Injury (%)	p-Value
Depression	68.46	53.28	< 0.0001*
PTSD	66.53	49.90	< 0.0001*

* An asterisk indicates that $p < 0.0001$, and the difference between the two groups was at least 2 percentage points.

TABLE 3.14

Predictors of Depression and PTSD Symptoms

Predictor	Depression				PTSD			
	Unadjusted		Adjusted		Unadjusted		Adjusted	
	β	p-value	β	p-value	β	p-value	β	p-value
Veteran has head injury	2.42	< 0.0001	0.12	0.0039	8.45	< 0.0001	1.44	< 0.0001
Total number of physical injuries	0.63	< 0.0001	0.04	< 0.0001	1.89	< 0.0001	0.12	0.0186
Total number of mental injuries	2.54	< 0.0001	2.05	< 0.0001	8.56	< 0.0001	7.07	< 0.0001
Total number of activities requiring assistance	0.88	< 0.0001	0.58	< 0.0001	2.52	< 0.0001	1.61	< 0.0001
Total number of WWP programs that the veteran participates in	0.33	< 0.0001	−0.05	0.0003	1.36	< 0.0001	0.07	0.3738
Hazardous drinking	0.75	< 0.0001	0.75	< 0.0001	4.42	< 0.0001	3.59	< 0.0001
Drug use	2.51	< 0.0001	0.85	< 0.0001	8.81	< 0.0001	2.55	< 0.0001

NOTE: The adjusted models also included adjustment for age, gender, educational attainment, race/ethnicity, marital status, and housing status. Full model results are presented in Appendix B.

TABLE 3.15

Predictors of Sleep Quality

Predictor	Bivariate (Unadjusted)		Adjusted	
	β	p-value	β	p-value
Veteran has head injury	1.44	< 0.0001	0.09	0.0848
Total number of physical injuries	0.41	< 0.0001	0.15	< 0.0001
Total number of mental injuries	1.28	< 0.0001	0.97	< 0.0001
Total number of activities requiring assistance	0.44	< 0.0001	0.27	< 0.0001
Total number of WWP programs that the veteran participates in	0.24	< 0.0001	0.01	0.3728
Hazardous drinking	0.57	< 0.0001	0.47	< 0.0001
Drug use	1.38	< 0.0001	0.42	< 0.0001

Substance Use

The survey asked respondents about their drinking and drug use. Hazardous drinking was measured with three questions from the Alcohol Use Disorders Identification Test – Concise (better known as the AUDIT-C) that ask about drinking frequency, quantity, and frequency of having six or more drinks. The scale ranges from 0 to 12, and a score of 3 or more for men and 2 or more for women was used to define hazardous drinking (Bradley et al., 2003; Bush et al., 1998). The Annual Warrior Survey also asked about drug use in the past year for multiple drug classes; for this analysis, we distinguished among marijuana use, opiate use, and other drug use, which included use of amphetamines, barbiturates, tranquilizers, cocaine, heroin, psychedelics, or other prescription or over-the-counter drugs neither prescribed nor used as intended. A greater share of those with a head injury than of those without a head injury reported marijuana use (21 percent versus 17 percent) and opiate use (11 percent versus 8 percent). Differences were not present for hazardous drinking or other drug use (Table 3.16).

Health Care Utilization, Access, and Barriers to Care

The Annual Warrior Survey asked respondents about their use of medical care and ease of accessing such care. As shown in Table 3.17, a greater share of those with a head injury than of those without a head injury had accessed medical care in the past three months (71 percent versus 66 percent), had sought mental health care (54 percent versus 44 percent), and had mental health pharmacotherapy (78 percent versus 73 percent). However, a greater share of those with a head injury also reported difficulty accessing mental health care (36 percent versus 28 percent) and physical health care (44 percent versus 33 percent).

TABLE 3.16

Prevalence of Hazardous Drinking and Drug Use Among WWP Survey Respondents, by Head Injury Status

Substance Use	With Head Injury (%)	Without Head Injury (%)	p-Value
Hazardous drinking	42.21	42.56	0.0125
Drug Use			
Marijuana	21.14	17.22	< 0.0001*
Opiates	11.11	8.25	< 0.0001*
Other	11.56	10.04	< 0.0001

* An asterisk indicates that $p < 0.0001$, and the difference between the two groups was at least 2 percentage points.

TABLE 3.17

Health Care Access Among WWP Survey Respondents, by Head Injury Status

Access	With Head Injury (%)	Without Head Injury (%)	p-Value
Accessed medical care in the past 3 months	71.17	66.00	< 0.0001*
Accessed mental health care in the past 3 months	53.61	43.84	< 0.0001*
Accessed mental health pharmacotherapy	77.75	73.43	< 0.0001*
Difficulty accessing mental health care	36.03	28.10	< 0.0001*
Difficulty accessing physical health care	43.63	33.48	< 0.0001*

* An asterisk indicates that $p < 0.0001$, and the difference between the two groups was at least 2 percentage points.

The survey also provided information about why veterans had difficulty accessing physical (Table 3.18) and mental (Table 3.19) health care. With respect to physical care, the barriers identified the most by those with a head injury were difficulty scheduling appointments (39 percent), difficulty getting referrals from VA (33 percent), and a lack of available VA specialty clinics (33 percent), all of which were greater than the share identified by those without a head injury (35 percent, 28 percent, and 27 percent, respectively). These outcomes may reflect that a smaller share of those without a head injury used VA for health care, as described earlier and presented in Table 3.5. The only barrier that was *less* common among those with a head injury relative to those without was having a personal schedule that conflicted with the hours of operation of VA health care facilities (27 percent of those with a head injury versus 32 percent of those without).

For mental health care, the barriers identified the most by those with a head injury were inconsistencies or lapses in treatment, feeling that treatment would bring up painful or traumatic memories, feeling uncomfortable with existing DoD or VA resources, and difficulty scheduling appointments (Table 3.19). Each of these barriers was endorsed by 32 percent of

TABLE 3.18

Barriers to Accessing Physical Health Care Among WWP Survey Respondents, by Head Injury Status

Barrier	With Head Injury (%)	Without Head Injury (%)	p-Value
Difficulty scheduling appointments	38.98	35.16	< 0.0001*
VA requirements made it difficult to get referrals to needed specialty treatment for physical problems	33.38	28.16	< 0.0001*
A lack of availability in VA specialty clinics (e.g., orthopedics, dental)	32.66	26.66	< 0.0001*
Inconsistent treatment or lapses in treatment (e.g., canceled appointments, had to switch providers)	29.82	25.12	< 0.0001*
Personal schedule (work, school, family responsibilities) conflicted with the hours of operation of VA health care facilities	27.16	31.74	< 0.0001*
Did not feel comfortable with existing resources within DoD or VA	20.97	17.59	< 0.0001*
A lack of resources for the veteran's physical health care problems in the relevant geographic area	18.18	13.69	< 0.0001*
Personal schedule (work, school, family responsibilities) conflicted with the hours of operation of non-VA health care facilities	15.54	16.85	0.0650
Could not afford copays or other costs not covered by health insurance	10.15	10.60	0.0483
Did not have health insurance to cover care for physical health problems	9.18	9.79	0.0292
Lacked transportation or the money to pay for transportation to get to health care services for physical health problems	8.83	6.99	< 0.0001
Concerned about losing job if asking for time off to receive health care services for physical health problems	8.50	9.05	0.0240
Did not know about existing resources available within DoD or VA	7.80	6.75	0.0002
A lack of nongovernment health care providers in the veteran's region who treat the relevant physical health problems	7.73	5.59	< 0.0001*
Did not have employer's support for taking the amount of time off needed to get to and receive health care services for physical health problems	6.14	5.78	0.2447
No peer support available	5.41	3.62	< 0.0001
Other reason(s) NOT marked above	30.08	30.52	0.1767

* An asterisk indicates that $p < 0.0001$, and the difference between the two groups was at least 2 percentage points.

TABLE 3.19

Barriers to Accessing Mental Health Care Among WWP Survey Respondents, by Head Injury Status

Barrier	With Head Injury (%)	Without Head Injury (%)	p-Value
Inconsistent treatment or lapses in treatment (e.g., canceled appointments, had to switch providers)	32.36	28.98	< 0.0001*
Felt that treatment might bring up painful or traumatic memories that the veteran wished to avoid	32.35	28.59	< 0.0001*
Did not feel comfortable with existing resources within DoD or VA	32.04	29.27	< 0.0001*
Difficulty scheduling appointments	31.82	29.05	< 0.0001*
Personal schedule (work, school, family responsibilities) conflicted with the hours of operation of VA health care facilities	30.49	35.33	< 0.0001*
A lack of VA mental health resources in the veteran's geographic area	26.58	20.76	< 0.0001*
VA requirements made it difficult to get referrals to needed specialty treatment for mental health problems	20.95	15.71	< 0.0001*
Felt that others would consider the veteran weak for seeking mental health treatment	17.90	17.42	0.2789
Concerned that future career plans would be jeopardized by seeking treatment	17.42	17.95	0.2027
Felt that the treatment was not appropriate for the symptoms	16.44	14.38	< 0.0001*
Felt that the treatment was not appropriate for the veteran's Operation Enduring Freedom, Operation Iraqi Freedom, or Operation New Dawn experience	16.19	10.00	< 0.0001*
Felt that peers or family would stigmatize the veteran for seeking mental health treatment	16.06	16.36	0.7553
Personal schedule (work, school, family responsibilities) conflicted with the hours of operation of non-VA health care facilities	15.92	17.11	0.0510
Lacked transportation or the money to pay for transportation to get to mental health care services	10.16	8.44	< 0.0001
Concerned about losing job if asking for time off to receive mental health care services	9.87	10.40	0.0756
No peer support available	9.78	7.41	< 0.0001*

Table 3.19—Continued

Barrier	With Head Injury (%)	Without Head Injury (%)	p-Value
A lack of nongovernment mental health care providers in the veteran's region	9.13	7.17	< 0.0001
Could not afford copays and other costs not covered by health insurance	7.56	7.21	0.1283
Did not know about existing resources available within DoD or VA	7.42	7.30	0.3824
Did not have employer's support for taking the amount of time off needed to get to and receive mental health care services	6.67	6.73	0.7415
Did not have health insurance that covers the veteran's mental health problems	6.49	7.12	0.1313
Other reason(s) NOT marked above	31.77	29.94	0.0031

* An asterisk indicates that $p < 0.0001$, and the difference between the two groups was at least 2 percentage points.

respondents with a head injury, which was significantly different from the share of those without a head injury who reported these barriers (29 percent). As with barriers to physical health care, the only mental health care barrier *less* common among those with a head injury than among those without was having a personal schedule that conflicted with the hours of operation of VA health care facilities (30 percent among those with a head injury versus 35 percent among those without).

Summary

The WWP Annual Warrior Survey is a rich source of information for identifying characteristics and potential needs of subpopulations, including veterans who experienced a head injury. In our analysis, respondents with a head injury differed in many ways from those without. For example, relative to those without a head injury, respondents with a head injury were more likely to be men, more likely to have been medically retired, and more likely to have served in the Army and Marine Corps. They were also more severely impaired (a larger share reported having higher VA and DoD Physical Evaluation Board disability ratings), had more physical and mental injuries, and had a greater reliance on caregivers. Although they were less likely to be employed, a comparable percentage of respondents with and without a head injury were enrolled in school, and more of those with a head injury who were enrolled were using government assistance to finance their education.

We also used the survey to identify the independent relationship between having a head injury and self-reported health, depression symptoms, PTSD symptoms, and sleep quality. After controlling for multiple factors, veterans with a head injury were more likely to report elevated PTSD and depression symptoms. Surprisingly, after controlling for such factors as physical and mental injuries and the need for caregiver support, those with a head injury indicated better self-reported health. There was no association between having a head injury and sleep quality after model adjustment.

Although they were more likely to be enrolled in VA health care, have Medicare, and have recently used medical and mental health care, WWP alumni with a head injury still faced multiple challenges accessing care. Breaks in the continuity of care and scheduling appointments presented challenges, as did distrust in government-sponsored services and a lack of available specialized VA services. And even though, compared with those without a head injury, those with a head injury had greater needs across multiple domains, utilization of WWP programs and services were relatively comparable between the two groups.

CHAPTER FOUR

Long-Term Experiences of Traumatic Brain Injury Among Veterans and Caregivers

In this chapter, we detail the methods and findings from our in-depth interviews with post-9/11 veterans and caregivers of veterans who suffered a TBI. The goal of this qualitative research was to complement the umbrella literature review (Chapter Two) and quantitative analysis (Chapter Three) with firsthand experiences and perspectives on the lived realities of aging with a TBI.

Approach to Interviews with Veterans and Caregivers

Sampling

WWP identified alumni who, in 2011 or earlier, self-reported a TBI, and WWP then sent an email to those individuals with a request to participate in an interview regarding their experiences living with TBI. Veterans could express interest in participating in an interview by calling or emailing the RAND team, or by signing up on a RAND website. Given the complications with classifying the severity of TBI, we did not ask veterans to specify whether they had a mild, moderate, or severe TBI (or multiple TBIs) as a condition of participation. Veterans were invited to ask their caregivers, if applicable, to participate in a separate interview about the caregiver's own experience. Caregivers were also able to reach out to RAND independently of the veteran for whom they provide care. Veterans and caregivers were each offered a $50 Amazon gift card to thank them for their time.

We scheduled interviews with all five veterans who telephoned the RAND team to express interest in an interview. We also responded to the first 50 veterans and caregivers who responded via email, which yielded another 27 interviews with veterans and eight interviews with caregivers. All interviews were conducted virtually between June and July 2021, during the coronavirus disease 2019 (COVID-19) pandemic.

Veterans were asked about their background in the military (e.g., years served, service branch). Veterans and caregivers were not asked about their demographic information, but we captured this information (e.g., race, gender) if it was freely offered by participants.

Interview Protocol

The interview protocol for veterans captured two overarching domains: (1) the diagnosis and treatment trajectories of those living with TBI and (2) the perceived support needs and suggested improvements to existing treatment programs. The interview protocol for caregivers centered on experiences of providing care and support for a veteran living with the impact of a TBI, the caregiver's own journey, concerns the caregiver has as the veteran ages, and the veteran's perceived support needs.

Interviews were conducted by phone or over Microsoft Teams based on the preference of the respondent. Interviewers recorded detailed notes (verbatim when possible) during interviews. In addition, we recorded all interviews following consent from respondents. The duration of the interviews ranged from 30 to 90 minutes, averaging around 45 minutes.

Data Analysis

We uploaded interview notes into Dedoose, a qualitative data analysis software that facilitates team-based coding (Dun & Bradstreet, undated). We developed a codebook based on the domains in the interview protocol (e.g., treatment-seeking behavior, quality of relationships, functional challenges), as well as topics of discussion that arose during interviews (e.g., volunteer work in one's community). Each set of notes was coded independently by a member of our research team trained in qualitative methods who also had sufficient topical expertise to identify key themes. The analysis followed Butler-Kisber's approach, in which we identified themes through repetition and specificity (i.e., similarities and differences among and within case studies) (Butler-Kisber, 2010), metaphors and analogies used, and existing knowledge of issues related to health service delivery in underserved populations (Ryan and Bernard, 2003). The initial analysis was then followed by a more fine-grained analysis, in which we identified and isolated specific phrases, terms, and ideas that veterans and caregivers used to convey their experiences.

Findings

Our final sample of 40 participants included five female veterans (or 15.6 percent, which is on par with the percentage of women among active-duty military personnel [15 percent]) (Parker, Cilluffo, and Stepler, 2017), 27 male veterans, and eight caregivers (including five female partners, one male partner, and two mothers of WWP alumni). All veterans but one (who sustained a TBI in a training exercise) sustained combat-related injuries during deployments between 2003 and 2015. All service branches were represented in the sample, including three from special operations forces, and the majority were Army veterans. Most TBIs were described as moderate or severe, although we did not ask veterans to provide medical documentation of TBI severity. The few who reported diagnosis of a mild TBI reported that they had sustained *multiple* mild TBIs. DoD data from August 2021 show that more than

80 percent of TBI cases were mild, while 11 percent were moderate and 2 percent were severe or penetrating (5 percent were not classifiable) (Military Health System, undated-a).

In broad strokes, the interviews revealed that veterans faced delays in the initial diagnosis of TBI; had co-occurring PTSD; endured additional physical injuries with persistent symptoms; and received combinations of care from DoD, the Veterans Health Administration (VHA), and community-based care, including through WWP's Warrior Care Network. The minority of veterans self-reported only minimal lasting consequences from their TBI and other injuries on their current health and well-being; the majority self-reported prolonged cognitive, mental health, functional, and physical hardships. Caregivers' experiences varied; for instance, only some received benefits and were engaged in caregiver networks. In this chapter, we describe these findings in more detail, beginning with how veterans described their initial injury or injuries; how and where they received care; the impact of comorbidities; their current health and well-being, relationships, employment, and educational experiences; caregiver experiences; and general support received and desired.

Traumatic Brain Injury in the Acute Phase

Diagnosis

Nearly every veteran reported delays in the diagnosis of TBI. There were several reasons for the delays, and some of those reasons, including a lack of universal screening for TBI in DoD until 2007, were echoed in interviews with subject-matter experts (see Chapter Seven). It was common to learn that veterans faced delays of several months and even years before being told they had a TBI. For example, as one veteran described,

> [My] TBI occurred in 2004, but I was not diagnosed until 2008. If it hadn't been for WWP and being in their Combat Stress [Recovery] Program, I would have never found out about TBIs since they were not a "thing" in 2004. There were no post-blast assessments.

In stating that TBIs were "not a 'thing,'" the veteran was not suggesting that TBIs did not exist but rather that regular screening for TBI did not become common practice until 2007. It is important to remember that many of the veterans in this sample were on the front lines during the initial stages of the Iraq and Afghanistan wars before standardized procedures were enacted. Even so, some in our interviews were skeptical that TBI screening assessments were being "taken seriously." Another veteran who suffered a TBI early on recounted,

> They kept me there [a military base in Germany] for maybe a week and they were like, "Well, we're just swamped, and we don't have the facilities." Then they sent me back. That's an experience I will never forget. I wouldn't wish it on anybody. Everything was new! Being on the first rotation and dealing with the first injuries, they tried to do as much as they could, but I don't think they were prepared for what was happening. Not only were they dealing with TBI—I mean, for every soldier that went out on the convoy,

if an IED went off—those things just shook you. It's like somebody took your head and shook it back and forth. Sometimes your ears would ring and after you go through that for a while—. But because you're a soldier, you can't complain, because if you do, it's "Suck it up! Don't be a wuss!" But all the same, they're going through what you're going through!

As a result, several veterans reported exposure to multiple blasts, often from IED explosions, in which they may have not lost consciousness or suffered other visible, physical injuries, leading them to continue on in their missions before enduring one definitive blast that sent them into a cascade of medical treatment, evaluation, and ultimately medical discharge from the military. One veteran reported having multiple concussions in jump school, including three concussions, or, as she put it, "three that I can *remember*. Three where I really got my bell rung." Another veteran described being concussed following a rocket attack and, months later, crash-landing in a Blackhawk, which caused another TBI and severe damage to her spine.

As described in Chapter Seven, diagnosing the severity of a TBI is hardly cut and dried. To veterans, the severity of the TBI (e.g., mild TBI) does not always reflect the intensity of the incident that caused the injury. For instance, as a veteran who was diagnosed with a mild TBI described,

> I was in the middle of a couple of explosions while following a tank, and then an IED went off. I got a pretty good bell ring there. We thought we were far enough away, but those explosions knock you out. If you have a door on your vehicle, the force of the explosion will shut the door. Since I was the medic for the group, they didn't do a whole lot. My ears weren't bleeding, and I could hear, so I just kept on going with the mission.

Others with moderate or severe TBI recalled vaguely remembering being in combat before waking up in a medical tent, or in Germany, realizing that they had lost consciousness for some time.

Veterans described that staying in combat zones and continuing to carry out the mission was of their own volition, "even after getting [their] bell rung." One special operations paratrooper who claimed to have had "repeated concussions for five years straight" was ultimately shot down in a helicopter and caught in heavy firefighting. He suffered from severe tinnitus, headaches, and vision loss, but when asked whether he was good enough to stay in the fight, he definitively replied yes. He added,

> I then went on to Afghanistan to prove that I could stay in. . . . I'd be trying to attack the enemy in their sleep, but I would have forgotten to wear one sock. The other guys were like, "You can't even read, man," but I was like, "I gotta stay in!"

Another veteran serving in the military police described getting hit with a "six-pack of explosives," causing a mild TBI that went unnoticed for a year. He redeployed, only to be sent home and medically retired after his commander said, "You've been in my office five times in the last 10 minutes to ask me the same question." But, to him, "if nothing was broken [after an attack], it was par for the course to say, 'Let's keep rocking and rolling!'" even though there were dozens of instances when he had to be sedated for migraines. "It was what it was," he added.

Staying in the fight, however, sometimes meant enduring one definitive blast causing other debilitating injuries (e.g., burns or damage to the skull, spine, or limbs) that sent the veteran away from the war zone, often to one of the U.S. military bases in Germany or the Walter Reed National Military Medical Center in Bethesda, Maryland. After evaluation and treatment, veterans were medically discharged and transferred to VA, where they were given a disability rating (seldom described as a straightforward process). And although many soon began new careers and started families after their service, all those interviewed gave the strong impression that their lives had changed in unpredictable ways since then. It is important to keep in mind that in no case was TBI the only ailment that veterans faced. Next, we explore common co-occurring health issues among this sample.

Common Co-Occurring Health Issues

Mental Health Issues

What makes the experience of TBI among veterans distinct from that among civilian populations is the often violent, traumatic incident that causes it. Such incidents often lead to co-occurring conditions, such as PTSD. The co-occurrence of TBI and PTSD is complicated by the fact that both share hallmark symptoms, such as irritability, apathy, concentration issues, and fatigue. A former Army Ranger said, "I have not met one infantry man that doesn't have PTSD," adding, "but their TBI gets overlooked [mistaken] for PTSD, and you send them to a support group and three-quarters of them are ticked off." Another veteran said that the "two conditions kind of overlap on each other and it's hard to tell them apart. I don't know which is which." While the two are intertwined, veterans described experiencing symptoms of PTSD, such as hypervigilance, reluctance to be in crowded spaces or in traffic, and paranoia. Furthermore, moral injury stemming from harm to children during combat caused three veterans in the sample significant grief, depression, and anxiety. Through prolonged therapy, these veterans were able to reprogram their memories of the traumatic events and restore function to their lives. Others had less-severe PTSD cases; as one veteran described,

> Not to dismiss what other people go through, but I just have nightmares. I try not to let whatever has happened affect me and my goals and what I want to do. I try to not hold onto those things. It would affect my personality. When I'm negative, I get depressed, and I'm not motivated to do much at all.

He laughed as he followed with, "My wife beats me into submission with positivity."

Interestingly, veterans also felt the same frustration echoed by clinicians that TBI and PTSD care are not addressed hand-in-hand. But the interviewees felt that the impact of their

TBI may have been downplayed when compared with the impact of and attention given to PTSD. As one veteran expressed,

> No one can say that this goes in the PTSD box, this goes in the TBI box. No one wants to blend the TBI and the PTSD clinic. These things are so interrelated, and we can't untangle it. Not everything I deal with is based on PTSD. My irritability levels are not just PTSD. It's unexplainable. You can't articulate the irritation. You can't control when that irritation is going to hit.

In another trend mirrored by clinicians (see Chapter Seven), symptoms of PTSD are often mistaken for TBI; that is, a veteran may feel that his symptoms are caused by TBI when they may actually be caused by PTSD. As one veteran expressed, "I had to get my VA care advocate involved because this doctor was just really mean and almost blatantly said that my TBI was not as severe as I seemed to think it was, and that it [my condition] was mostly PTSD-related." Although PTSD is arguably no longer as stigmatized as it has been in recent years, it is possible that there is a reluctance among veterans to ascribe their symptoms to PTSD, and it is also possible that, through delay and misdiagnoses, a veteran's TBI symptoms could be more persistent than anticipated.

Nearly every veteran in this interview sample reported having PTSD, and they described the symptoms of the condition coming in waves. For example, a veteran who was not medically discharged until 2012 described that he "got diagnosed with PTSD in 2003 and didn't even know that until 2007." He continued, "I didn't have any effects until a few years after, and then my wife and I were out one night, started drinking, and well, I got myself thrown in jail. I got out and started treatment for PTSD. Now all I can do is live my life as best I can."

Veterans also reported having depression and anxiety. During interviews, some recalled adverse childhood experiences, such as violence, that had resurfaced because of PTSD and TBI. One veteran spoke at length about this issue and how he struggles to manage his emotions in order to navigate everyday life and his relationships. Depression and suicidal ideation were compounded by challenges in navigating day-to-day life. A veteran who had enrolled in a master's program said that he disenrolled after getting Cs. As he described it,

> I needed more than just more time to take a test. I had problems forming sentences. I couldn't remember stuff. Even reading text on a white paper or the light of a computer screen just hurt. I had to get specialized lenses because my brain was different. The words on the paper look like they're moving. It made me want to fall asleep. I was having too many challenges and not enough tools.

After failing at the master's program, the veteran said that he "went into a serious depression. I was suicidal. It was a big struggle." Other veterans described more-generalized depression and anxiety brought on by a "flare up" of physical symptoms or when one's "body is not cooperating to get done what needs to get done."

Substance Use

This subsample of veterans with TBI reported previous or current alcohol and substance use, including daily use. For example, some described using alcohol in the military but not being discharged as a result:

> They didn't want to lose an asset. I was an alcoholic to recover from all the other issues. They never said, "You might have PTSD or something else going on." When it was egg on their face, that's when they stopped, but as long as I was doing my job, there was no problem.

As relayed by this veteran, alcohol use was an antidote to his PTSD, but even though he was on active duty, the military did not provide the needed diagnosis or treatment. Another veteran recounted giving up alcohol after his wife issued an ultimatum. A few reported using cannabis daily to cope with PTSD. Others battled addiction to pain medicine. Regardless of whether they were using alcohol or drugs, many veterans described auto accidents, physical accidents, and the wake of destruction that resulted. They had many friends who wound up dead, including by suicide. Knowledge of this possibility eventually affected at least one veteran:

> It took me a while to get treatment. It took me getting into trouble quite a bit before I could get treatment, and I came home to live at home with my mom and dad. I was getting in and out of trouble and had a couple of [convictions for driving under the influence]. That's what got me to where I had to do something or enjoy my life as an inmate. I went into intensive inpatient treatment at the VA. Then my case manager for VA told me about WWP.

That veteran began participating in services with WWP in about 2008 or 2009 and was not using alcohol at the time of the interview. There were also success stories of gaining sobriety from opioids, but for at least one veteran, that came on the heels of being hospitalized for a serious accident while high.

Only two veterans reported presently using cannabis regularly, but several more spoke of having problematic substance and alcohol use in their past. Those problems added a layer of complexity to seeking care for their complex array of additional mental and physical health disorders.

Co-Occurring Physical Health Issues

As noted by our interviewees, the diagnosis of a TBI often came in tandem with obvious physical (i.e., not invisible) wounds of war, such as spine injuries, broken pelvic bones, extreme migraines, and the degradation and destruction of the senses. Some veterans have had to learn how to walk again while dealing with their TBI, and others developed coping strategies for the loss of functionality. A former Army Ranger who endured the explosion of a 1,000-pound IED laced with a chemical agent described his "dizzy spells, nerve damage, incontinence and catheter, skin breakouts, PTSD that is off the charts, severe tinnitus, neck pain, bloody nose, concentration issues, bruxism, migraines, severe pain, and fatigue."

Many veterans with TBI experience hearing loss in one or both ears. One veteran who was "mechanically deaf" in the left ear and experienced "really bad tinnitus" in the right ear described his condition as follows: "It's hard for me to hear when people are saying stuff to me. So, I have people write stuff and read while they say it. I have an entire adaptive system around not being able to hear correctly to help me understand what people say." Tinnitus also was often reported as an irritating and debilitating comorbidity.

Seizures were also common among veterans with more-severe TBIs. Seizure types include simple, partial seizures (non-epileptic seizures) and repeated grand mal seizures (referred to as generalized tonic-clonic seizures). These not only are harmful physically and emotionally to the veterans but also place a strain on caregivers:

> I didn't get a handbook on caregiving, but there's definitely no guidance on how to help non-epileptic seizures. We had gone to the ER [emergency room] so many times to the point that they said, "Don't come back unless he hurts himself while having a seizure." No one listened to me as a spouse when I said what worked and what didn't . . . . In the humidity, it's rough, but overall, a lot better. He went from 2015–16, he was having three to four seizures a day; they could be in spurts for 20 minutes, but the whole episode would last 2.5 hours, but he'd also be seizing in his sleep. We were lucky if he didn't seize for a day or two. And now we're kind of at a point where he can go a couple of weeks without a seizure. He seized on the Fourth of July because neighbors were lighting fireworks. Because he doesn't have the seizures as often, the recovery period is almost just as long as it used to be."

Even when seizures become less frequent, they can still significantly decrease quality of life for the veteran and caregiver. This wife also revealed something that was far too common across all conditions: caregivers (and veterans) not feeling heard in encounters with medical providers.

Migraines were also a chief complaint among those with several moderate or severe TBIs. Veterans tried to describe the pain levels of a migraine. In fact, one veteran went to the ER after cutting his finger with a table saw in the days following the interview. He followed up over email, writing,

> When we went to urgent care, nurse took my blood pressure (not that elevated) and cleaned the cut. It hurt some, but I didn't react too much. Alarmed, she said, "Mr. ——, can you feel this?" I said, "Yep. Not great, but still not close to my migraines."

Another veteran relayed a collection of symptoms that extends from migraines to the other senses, as he occasionally sees aura (stars) and has lost vision on the left side of both eyes (ongoing since 2003), and he has also experienced frequent headaches, some short-term memory loss, and tinnitus. He added,

> I get headaches 24/7. Pain level is at a nine every day. I got used to it, but when it goes up to a 10, that's what I'm not used to and morphine is the only thing that helps. But, I want to find something else. . . . I go to Polytrauma [the VA's Polytrauma/TBI System of Care]

for neck pain, do physical therapy, but it's not helping. It only loosens for an hour and then it's back the way it is. I told my doctor, if I can't walk, then do surgery. If I can still walk, then let's do more conservative-type steps.

Vision impairment, ranging from light sensitivity to very limited sight, was also common in this sample. In some instances, the severity can change over time, as recounted by one veteran:

I got blown up at least 35 times . . . . There's something wrong with the wiring that goes from the brain to the eye. I have no peripheral vision, and depth perception is extremely obscured. It's been like that since 2005 and has just been getting progressively worse.

Other veterans gave up their driver's license voluntarily to avoid putting others at risk. Hence, comorbidities can greatly affect activities of daily life among veterans with a TBI.

As noted earlier, a TBI seldom occurs in isolation; hence, while veterans struggled with a TBI diagnosis, they also faced a complex constellation of co-occurring physical and mental health disorders. Receiving treatment for these conditions in the years following discharge from the military was a consistently complicated process that involved several care transitions without a guarantee of a warm or effective handoff throughout those transitions.

Accessing Care

Nearly every veteran in this sample sought care from multiple health care systems and in locations across the United States for treatment of their TBI, as well as for the variety of physical and mental health issues that commonly co-occur with TBI. Many veterans with TBI described the process of being transported from the battlefield to Germany for immediate care and then to the Walter Reed National Military Medical Center for more-extensive acute care. Acute care was described as treatment for serious physical injuries rather than care for the chronic conditions that often come with being a wounded warrior (e.g., chronic pain, PTSD, and the long-term impacts of TBI). Some veterans categorized this time as the period before medical retirement, which some felt they were forced into. As a veteran with a decades-long tenure in the military described, "My last posting was in Iraq as a senior squad leader. We were there for seven months before I got injured, and that put me in a three-year medical hold status while they tried everything to get me back to being recovered before they put me out to pasture."

Following medical discharge, every veteran in the sample sought care at VA either exclusively or in conjunction with community-based care. Despite the fact that all of the veterans in the sample had polytraumas, only a few in the sample received care in one of VA's five Polytrauma Transitional Rehabilitation Program sites. Those who did were generally satisfied with the level of care that they received. As one veteran noted,

I was put into the VA polytrauma system in 2012 after a couple of years of trying to figure out stuff. Polytrauma helped with lots of little things, like light sensitivity. I hadn't gone to a doctor for little things like that, I only went for the big problems. I was in poly for about a year and sent to the in-residence TBI program, which was for both TBI and PTSD because they couldn't separate them. That connected me to WWP.

This veteran went on to describe enrolling in early WWP programming. At the time, WWP offered a year-long in-person program that offered, as the veteran described, "counseling, individual health, wellness, linkages to the right specialist." WWP also helped him get his medical disability rating increased and his retirement backdated. Finally, this veteran described receiving care through WWP's Warrior Care Network to "focus on coping skills and not treatment."

Another veteran had been to four different VA sites (including one that he "won't send anyone to"). His main issue was the narrower focus on treating PTSD. He added,

They had good PTSD docs, but they wanted to see the entire world as a PTSD problem. I'd tell them, "No, I have a TBI. Look here." You need someone who can see the whole, holistic set of factors. The VAs don't talk to each other. Everyone wants to b---- about the DoD not talking to each other, but the VA is worse!

The veteran ultimately received care at a VA polytrauma site. He explained,

They sat me down and talked to me about what I could do. They had a multidisciplinary team—[occupational therapy, physical therapy], speech therapy, neurology, vision specialists, and they sent me to an eye hospital that took in veterans. That VA was great.

Veterans who were unable to access care at a VA polytrauma site reported that the quality of care at VA was inconsistent. This finding is not altogether surprising given our sample of post-9/11 veterans, and especially a sample that was eventually linked to care through WWP (i.e., a group of veterans who had sought care and support outside of VA).

It was common for veterans to describe seeing a specialist within VA but not having much success in addressing their condition. One veteran who had experienced a rocket attack during Operation Enduring Freedom said, "I was seeing a not-so-good neurologist in the VA. After six months, he said, 'I don't know how to take care of you, goodbye. I don't deal with headaches.'" The veteran eventually sought care at a TBI-specific community-based program for balance, visual, and speech therapy. He then returned to VA to maintain occupational, physical, and speech therapy but was "given a few Sudoku games and told, 'See you later,' and some speech therapy over the phone." He has since sought care from a community-based neurologist (covered by TRICARE) who is treating damage to the occipital and frontal lobes of the brain, which the neurologist linked to speech, hearing, vision, and pain issues. In addition, this veteran had found pain relief in hyperbaric oxygen therapy, despite its inconclusive effectiveness in the literature, but was unable to continue it because of prohibitively high out-of-pocket costs. Although each veteran's journey is unique, this narrative was indicative of the involved and lengthy process of receiving care.

Several veterans in the sample indicated that the care they received at VA was "fantastic" (especially at VA polytrauma sites) and that they had "never had a problem." But, as noted earlier, veterans in this sample were frustrated that individual VA sites "don't talk to each other," which, interestingly, was echoed by clinicians. Some veterans gave up on driving long distances to the nearest VA, and others muscled through the nearly 200 miles roundtrip to receive specialty care. For veterans seeking treatment for co-occurring PTSD, some resented being seen by mental and behavioral health specialists who were naïve to the challenges of deployment and combat. Others were frustrated by group therapy sessions in which "there were other guys who really didn't have tough traumas." And the need for referrals to seek community-based care was also a source of frustration. One veteran who suffered from debilitating migraines and chronic pain described how VA could be doing more to promote complementary and alternative medicine:

> This is where the VA or TRICARE could be doing more [to cover] chiropractors, acupuncture, all of these alternative options, especially given the fact that they no longer give out pain medication. They should be highly encouraging their members to take up these alternative therapies. One VA established a pain clinic with chiropractors, acupuncture, but it took two hours to get there. We would have literally had to move. So, we pay out of pocket for the chiropractor. It's frustrating.

Despite the barrage of complaints about access to and quality of care, a few veterans were satisfied with the care that they received immediately following and in the first few years after their TBI diagnosis. One veteran made a point of saying, "I will openly tell you that I think the Army did well by me." But, as was too often the case, persistent health challenges meant that veterans would remain within these various complex systems of care.

Traumatic Brain Injury in the Post-Acute Phase

Current Health and Well-Being

When asked about their current health and well-being several years after their injuries, veterans provided a variety of responses. All were still managing chronic conditions, but overall health, well-being, and functionality differed substantially across the sample. Several veterans felt that they were able to manage their health and well-being, but many still felt plagued by physiological, physical, and mental health issues.

With respect to ongoing health issues, some spoke of metabolic disorders, such as diabetes, or struggled with weight gain. Others cited chronic pain and ongoing injuries. As one veteran explained,

> I'm stuck in neutral with internal injuries. I'm at home twiddling my thumbs. I wish I had lost a limb so that I could be fixed. I have useless limbs because they are still attached to my body. I have no ligaments in my shins, bad Achilles tendons, and I wear splints. All

of this simply because of my military service. My legs are less than useless, but they're attached to my body. I'll pull into a handicap spot with a cane or a walker and people will look at me, but they can't see the titanium in my body.

Hearing and vision loss—or, as one veteran put it, being "half blind and half deaf"—were also common complaints. Another veteran added, "My ears have not stopped ringing. My neck still hurts. I have extreme sensitivity to light. . . . I feel like I'm from a different planet." Several veterans spoke of balance issues. In addition, a few reported that damage to the hypothalamus incurred through the TBI created a hormonal imbalance, such as low testosterone.

But, by far, veterans reported memory loss and reduced cognitive function as their chief complaints. A veteran described a recurring situation in which he tells his wife that he will run errands for the family, and then he will

> drive to Dollar General, Lowe's, or Food Lion, but I'll get there and forget what the hell I'm there for. I'll go with a list but forget to look at it and come home with tons of other stuff. We're doing as much as we can for me to remain functioning and independent, but then we deal with stuff like that.

Other veterans described being frustrated by stuttering or not being able to "find the right words." For some, this meant being "not as mentally with it as I used to be, but it hasn't been a dramatic downfall, except that sometimes I feel more forgetful." For several veterans, the cognitive issues were coupled with physical challenges; as one veteran noted, "I can't move fluidly through society." Another veteran said,

> I still have problems with losing track of a conversation. Sometimes my speech is slurred or my vocabulary is gone, and I'm misusing words now. I still have vestibular issues from time to time. I've actually lost my balance, hit my head, had another concussion. When the Botox cycle is coming to an end, it gets harder to control the headaches. I had to go to the ER twice this past month.

Despite some veterans having seemingly overwhelming health issues, several displayed a positive outlook. One summarized his current health as follows:

> Things now are better. Every now and then, I still have an issue with remembering words or my speech doesn't flow as well as I would want it to. My balance is still horrible, so I cannot walk heel-to-toe. They told me that if I were ever to get a sobriety test, I would fail every time. I still have astigmatism, my chronic, constant headaches that have never gone away. But, you know, at this point, I'm so used to it that I won't even notice that they're there unless I think about it. It's the same with the tinnitus; if I don't think about it, I don't notice it. Sometimes the tinnitus will go from sounding like a summer night with crickets and then every once in a while, it'll change to a loud whistle and *that* one you can't ignore.

In addition to describing memory loss, many veterans reported persistent migraines and intense headaches. One veteran noted, "The first five years were pretty much a nightmare.

They were generally terrible. Now, it's only bad when the barometric pressure rolls in. But the memory loss is still there, which is pretty common, but it depends; there's no rhyme or reason to it."

For several veterans in the sample, PTSD remains a persistent challenge. For example, some described having difficulty in public spaces, while others who had found effective treatment reported that their PTSD symptoms had improved. One interviewee said that the "PTSD is much better. I can go to the store without having to go hide. When I first got back, I couldn't go to the store. Now I'm not happy about going, but it's okay, even if I still have hypervigilance." Another described that his once-monthly migraines were compounded by a lack of sleep, which was caused by PTSD-related nightmares. Veterans poignantly described these experiences as "*normal* PTSD stuff." One veteran said, "I break out in a cold sweat, and my wife kicks me away." He added that he is "doing mentally much better ten years later" and is able to "work out twice a day three days a week and once on the other days."

Overall, veterans with TBI each relayed many current health challenges across multiple domains with varying degrees of progress following the acute phases of their injuries. In the next section, we briefly explore care-seeking and treatment received for present-day health challenges among veterans.

Current Treatment

In descriptions of their current treatment, veterans with TBI described a combination of maintenance efforts and levels of satisfaction with their options. Veterans reported seeking care within the VA system, from community-based care, and through WWP's Warrior Care Network sites. Although veterans commonly used and often praised the VA Polytrauma/TBI System of Care, their feelings about the VA system tended to be negative (although not exclusively so). It was not the focus of this study to evaluate programs, but all veterans who sought care for PTSD and TBI through Warrior Care Network intensive outpatient settings reported experiencing success—or, as one veteran who struggled with moral injury described, "being able to move past stuck points."

Veterans did not report seeking extensive care to maintain their physical health, which was perhaps the result of their current health status, a lack of available care options, or the care they had received in prior years. Rather, many were not currently participating in regular treatment. For example, one veteran said that he is "not seeking any treatment. I go to the VA for annual checkups, dentist, and eyes. Healthwise, I'm good. Because of the [COVID-19] pandemic, I put on some weight, but short of that, everything is fine." Others described finding relief in treatments for which the evidence base does not definitively show effectiveness, such as using an Alpha-Stim electrotherapy machine or undergoing hyperbaric oxygen therapy. Several veterans reported finding relief for their migraines from Botox injections, which have become easier to access in recent years. Additionally, many emphasized that regular exercise was important for their physical health, though it is not a form of treatment. Overall, the statements by veterans in this sample indicated that the bulk of their physical medical treatment was behind them, but they nevertheless shared common forms of maintenance.

However, many spoke at greater length about their mental health treatment. Given the depth of their psychological challenges, many veterans still participated in treatment for PTSD. As one veteran described,

> I go to the psychiatrist at the VA, and she helps me with the PTSD. I have problems sleep-ing and deal with nightmares. As far as the TBI, I haven't gotten too much treatment aside from the headaches. They did memory tests and stuff when they initially diagnosed me but nothing after that.

As he described, this veteran received therapy for PTSD, but he was not receiving care for his perceived cognitive deficits.

Other veterans expressed dissatisfaction with their treatment. For example, one veteran relayed,

> I'm still in active therapy for PTSD, and I have a counselor and a [nurse practitioner] in psychology, but he's worthless. He just makes sure I'm breathing and not going to kill anybody or myself. I'd rather talk to a robot. COVID was a blessing because I didn't have to go in and see him.

Others described less-intensive supportive treatment. One interviewee said, "For con-tinuous care, I'm part of Wounded Warrior Project's Independence Program. The program connects me with people who keep me straight on certain things, like life coaches to make sure I'm getting stuff done." This veteran had reached a point when maintenance was the primary need of his mental health program. This was not the norm though, and many veter-ans described participating in more-active treatment to assist them with the challenges that remained for their psychological well-being.

Challenges Associated with Traumatic Brain Injury

Changes to Identity

The transition from service member to veteran can create a cascade of challenges related to work, relationships, and sense of purpose. Most of the veterans in this sample were medically discharged before they had intended to separate from the military, and they spoke emotion-ally about the sudden loss of their military identities. A veteran said,

> From day one, once I got that non-deployable status, I found out I didn't mean s--- any-more. It was a very dehumanizing experience. Losing your entire identity, all that pain. If I wasn't a logical person, I can't imagine where I'd be right now.

The added challenge of having ongoing health issues and new limitations of body and mind led veterans to change how they viewed themselves. This was particularly pronounced among veterans of U.S. Army Special Forces and other special operations forces (e.g., Navy SEALs). As expressed by a Green Beret, "I was a combat helicopter pilot, top of my field, endurance for days, spoke several languages. Now, trying to problem solve, I just get exhausted, and I feel overwhelmed." An Army Ranger with young triplets at home poignantly described that he has to have his children wear sneakers with Velcro fastenings because he has difficulty tying shoelaces. He added, "The simplest things I won't be able to do, and then I get frustrated. I used to be a super *stud* and now I'm a super *dud*. . . . I went from being a superstar Army Ranger to being a guy who the VA said was unemployable." As a result of the damage from TBI (and possibly other injuries), many veterans lost the foundation to their sense of self. That shook many to their core.

In response, some veterans rebuilt themselves with a new view of who they were. It often began with a focus on family. One said,

> There's only one thing you can't get back and that's time. I just want my time moving forward as the best me for my family so that I can enjoy everything. I've earned that . . . . I need to be the best me going forward for this family. At the end of this month, I'll become a grandpa! At 44!

This veteran learned how to focus on the present through enjoyment of his family and to be the best version of himself. Another veteran displayed a combination of self-appreciation and humor:

> I don't know what kind of person I would be without all of those experiences, but I would probably be less interesting. I would have less stories to tell. I like me, who I am now. I don't know if I would be more motivated to do some of the things that I'm doing. I think everything that has happened has shaped me into who I am. I definitely still have short-term memory loss. She [my wife] very kindly reminds me. My kids don't know that very well though, and they will remind me with a little more aggression, so we write things down and update calendars as needed.

Regardless of the stage of their identity development, the challenges were profound for the veterans, as summarized in one's reflection that "I want to be a normal guy, whatever that is. I've just experienced so much. I've seen the worst of humanity." As a result of all they've been through—deployment, combat, trauma, TBI, other injuries—their understanding of what is normal has been uprooted. Rebuilding their identity is an enormous undertaking compounded by TBI.

Employment and Education

The veterans we interviewed had both positive and negative experiences with education and employment since experiencing TBI in the military. Several obtained their bachelor's and master's degrees, including with assistance from WWP. For example, WWP programming helped participants earn college credits and placed them into a career-relevant job. Another person mentioned the transition training academy that helped him get into his career, but the program no longer exists. Unfortunately, some people with TBI struggled academically because of difficulties with concentration and memory. Others benefited from academic accommodations that included receiving printed material (as opposed to reading on computer screens) and extensions on assignments when needed. Those accommodations could be coordinated by the campus Student Veteran Administration; as one veteran described, "The woman who ran it was in a car accident, so she understood. I could read something five times and only remember two paragraphs. She got me a notetaker and into classrooms [with professors who were supportive]." These experiences demonstrated ways that, with the proper supports, veterans with TBI could succeed academically.

Similarly, many veterans related positive work experiences that often involved understanding colleagues. One veteran described the supportive environment in his service industry job, where he fit well with his co-workers, including his supervisors. They shared the same temperament, and employees could discuss issues with the bosses. This helped his comfort and confidence, particularly with regard to making mistakes and being forgetful—challenges from his TBI. Other veterans detailed their strategies for addressing memory issues, such as frequently taking notes and maintaining a calendar. Nevertheless, some struggled at work and left their jobs. As one described,

> I would be going through training and stuff like that, and I would remember it for a little while and I might go back two days after that and be sitting there like, "Okay, I gotta do—what I gotta do?" I wrote a lot of notes, and I used to have to go back to them. I just recently resigned from my job because I really couldn't keep up. I couldn't sit for a long period of a time because of my neck and back, and it was very fast-paced, and you had to remember a thousand passwords and log into a lot of computer programs, and it just got overwhelming.

Many veterans reported having full-time employment, but TBI often adds challenges to being successful at work, especially from issues with memory and hearing. Some in high-ranking professions described a bias or stigma against combat veterans with TBI. One veteran recalled, "I remember when I told people at work that I have TBI, people started talking louder."

Unfortunately, many veterans with TBI were unable to maintain their jobs, including one who was unable "to keep a job for more than six months." Another who had recently finished college was struggling to find full-time employment. He explained, "If I apply and I tell people I need accommodations, then I don't get a call back." Both the positive and negative experiences in school and jobs revealed the importance of finding a supportive and understanding fit. Although this may be true for people in general, it seems especially the case for veterans with TBI.

Romantic Relationships

For some veterans with TBI, their romantic relationships were sources of strength in dealing with their injuries and trauma. These veterans relied on their partners for emotional support and for assistance in taking physical care of themselves, and they appreciated their partners' patience while working through TBI-related cognitive issues. These circumstances also taxed some relationships, and at the time of the interviews, some were separated from their partners or were in the process of finalizing a divorce. All described some degree of difficulty in having a relationship in which one partner has persistent health challenges.

In speaking of his relationship's success, one veteran talked about being persistent, adding, "We've done therapy, which has helped a little, and committed to staying together. She knows what I went through. It's been a lot of work and forgiveness." Another veteran said that getting married "gave me purpose." A wife of a veteran with TBI described feeling fulfilled by being able to provide care and cook meals while her husband redeveloped his cognitive skills. Thus, romantic relationships could be strengthened or serve as a source of stability during this period.

On the other hand, many romantic relationships worsened over time. The stresses and issues sometimes became too much for a partner to handle. "Our divorce will be final next month," one veteran said in a somber tone, adding, "She was very supportive through the initial injury and the aftermath, and at some point, she just got to the point where it was too much to remember all my crap and remind me to do everything and keep up with kids and everything else." Several veterans relayed that their anger management issues contributed to their relationships breaking apart, although they took responsibility for that to varying degrees. One veteran recounted, "I got divorced after the explosion. I had some anger issues, and she just wasn't willing to help me figure it out. She didn't know what to do, so she left." In sum, the stresses from these veterans' injuries, including TBI, and the frequent related anger issues were too much for some romantic relationships to survive.

Additional Stress

As with all people, veterans with TBI have additional stressors in life that affect their health and well-being. For example, being a parent is not easy for anyone, and the trauma related to deployment and the subsequent injury can add to that difficulty. One veteran said that he and his wife "have four children, and our 17-year-old [the youngest] is the only one [still] here. It's [recently] been easier to spend time with him. We had a strained relationship because I wasn't home and then when I was home, I wasn't available." He further described that his career as an analyst for a government contractor requires him to review disturbing images that he described as "traumatic." Veterans and caregivers also described the need to care for children and grandchildren who may have health issues of their own. Financial issues, sometimes incurred through self-described "mistakes," were an additional source of strain. Furthermore, life events can disrupt the hard-won balance that veterans may have over their symptoms, as was the case with a veteran who was selling her house, and the stress upset work she had done to accept and manage her health.

Prior life trauma also poses challenges that can be exacerbated by TBI. For example, one veteran who thought he had come to terms with his childhood abuse described his "reactive attachment disorder from a violent childhood. I dealt with it, but it came back out through the TBI." This was echoed by another veteran who spoke of repeated trauma during her childhood and military sexual trauma during her time in the service. Thus, in addition to the complex health challenges posed by TBI, veterans face many of the same stressors that are common in life. However, TBI can change the nature of those pressures and make coping with them that much more difficult.

Coping Strategies and Support Received

Veterans described an array of strategies for coping with their injuries. Some expressed that they had to develop a new sense of their capabilities; one stated, "At this point, it'll just mean coming to a general understanding of what it is. Speech, balance, memory—establishing a new normal." This coping strategy helped some veterans adjust their expectations of what they were capable of and how life would be. This allowed some to be practical about their lives; as one noted, "I focus on functionality and not on feeling good. Doing the things I need to do to be successful to have my career." The coping mechanism allowed others to live life in the here and now. A common approach among the veterans was to remind themselves that many others had it worse. One veteran stated, "I didn't complain. Everyone has their own injuries and things going on in your life, and they don't want to hear what you have to say." That veteran tried to stay positive in life and earned a bachelor's and master's degree despite doctors being pessimistic about recovery. Some veterans used their faith as a foundation, expressing the belief that "God had a purpose and everything worked out okay." Others moved into a state of acceptance; as one person said, "I know there is no medical cure for TBI, only management. I had to come to accept that." Each of these approaches reflected an outlook that enabled the veterans to identify the positive in their lives and build on it.

Other methods for coping were more specific to the veterans' injuries. For some, staying physically active was an important coping strategy. This could take the form of outdoor activities (e.g., hunting, camping), regular exercise, or athletic competition. One veteran described not knowing whether the benefits were from being "a stress reliever or the endorphins, but once I started really working out a lot, it helped with everything." Those who needed special equipment to meet their needs obtained them through purchase or donation. For pain management, some practiced complementary or alternative medicine, such as yoga, acupuncture (and other traditional Chinese medicine), and Alpha-Stim electrotherapy. Some veterans recognized the connection between the physical and the psychological: "I do so much mind-body stuff. It helps!" For others, immersing themselves in activities with deep focus (e.g., beekeeping, shooting firearms or arrows) provided relief because the concentration was so great that they would lose track of time. They could not say whether it was the focus or the controlling of actions (e.g., breathing, panic) that helped them reset.

TBI also caused cognitive damage, and veterans adapted to their new needs. As previously detailed, they had to develop techniques at home and work to compensate for their memory challenges. Coping skills could also involve an overall approach to life; as one veteran described, "I have to slow the pace down. I can't be at the operational pace. Just focus on that one thing. If you try to do too many things, you're setting yourself up to fail." This last statement was also reflective of the larger coping mechanism of veterans adjusting their expectations of themselves—being realistic about their new normal and finding ways to achieve it.

Veterans with TBI described a variety of sources that currently provide support. They frequently mentioned family and friends who helped with care and handling life; one veteran noted, "Family support is really big for me, especially in the first few years where I was entirely dependent on their help." When they achieved more stability in their life, the veterans appreciated friends who simply "got them out of the house" for an afternoon. Longer stretches of time away can be important too, and many valued outdoor activities with other veterans. This "adventure therapy" included camping, hunting, and road trips. WWP has been instrumental in support by offering outdoor programs, such as Project Odyssey; virtual events during the COVID-19 pandemic, including events with caregivers; and other activities, such as cooking classes, fishing trips, online yoga classes, and regional peer groups. One veteran stated, "WWP has done more for me than the military and the VA. They have, literally and figuratively." Some veterans also participated in telehealth that included psychotherapy, wellness groups, and art therapy. For some veterans, work has been a great source of support, often providing the meaning and satisfaction that can come from the right job. In addition, veterans indicated that colleagues have been helpful; as one veteran related,

> When I told them about it [the TBI], they were really cool about it. They never stopped seeing how they could help out. I only started working there in March, so to tell them I need time off for major surgery, most places would say, "it was a fun run while it lasted." They're willing to work with me when I'm ready to get back.

Other veterans mentioned that colleagues would help with notetaking and adapt their communication to accommodate needs. For veterans with TBI, ongoing support is crucial. They find it in many different relationships and situations as people find ways to value them and assist them as they navigate the world.

Service to Others

Many veterans with TBI spoke of the service they provided to other veterans with TBI. Some did so through informal interactions and relationships, while others went so far as to establish nonprofit organizations. Often, the desire to help others grew from their own struggles, whether with mental health, physical health, or navigating VA. One interviewee noted, "The VA looks at people as being a number and not a person. When you first get out, that's not a good feeling. I try to help other wounded warriors and guide and mentor them. I give them help and information. I try to teach others." Another veteran with TBI who established a nonprofit organization that holds several events each year for veterans explained, "It really helped me not be as bitter. . . . For the first couple years, I'd get so angry about how I felt I was treated, so it was tough. Being able to work through that has been so helpful. It makes you feel good. It's amazing how people who have next to nothing will give that last little bit."

For many, being of service to others, including those struggling with their own TBI, has been a source of great self-worth. Many veterans' groups are dominated by white men, so a need exists for more women and people of color. As a result, some veterans made the extra effort to reach out to fellow veterans of color. As one described, "I mentor him and tell him it's [the treatment of veterans of color in veterans' groups] not personal; he's gotta work through it." The stories of service that were relayed by the veterans suggest that giving back to others is central to the survival of the community and also helps heal the mentor.

Concerns About the Future

Because of their injury, veterans with TBI had apprehensions about their long-term prospects related to health and quality of life. For starters, veterans often did not receive guidance about their future; one learned that he would "do all the recovery in the first two years, and then it's just going to be what it is." Veterans explained that, beyond that, they had a lack of information about how their health would progress or their needs change. Several expressed concerns about premature death, and one was living with the belief that "I could die any day. The VA said I could drop dead anytime." The majority, however, expressed concerns about declines in brain functioning, having been warned about developing Parkinson's disease, dementia, and early-onset Alzheimer's after living with memory-related issues for several years. One veteran explained,

> They told me about early-onset Alzheimer's as soon as I was diagnosed with the TBI. It was gut-wrenching. It was just like I got cancer or something. I was kinda down for a while, but I never told anybody. I told my wife, but telling her and actually seeing the results now are like day and night. Back when they told me, it was just like, "When I get older, I'm gonna start feeling these effects." Well, they don't tell you that it might be even earlier than you'd expect. They don't really tell you a specific time. It bothered me, but I was still fairly young back then. As far as my memory, it didn't bother me so much, but now I am really seeing what they were talking about.

Coinciding with the fears about their health was the continued skepticism about the quality of care provided by VA. Some veterans were even still battling with VA over the proper diagnosis of their TBI, so some did not trust the system as a whole or its doctors to provide the health care that they needed. In addition, many veterans did not live near the major VA centers. One caregiver explained, "And what are the long-term effects of war on his body? Is he going to have adequate care going forward? Our VA is a little VA that doesn't have all the services he needs. We have to fight for everything here." The ramifications of the health challenges extend throughout life.

Other veterans described a feeling of acceptance over the future and a sense of grace for where they were. One veteran added,

> Today I'm feeling pretty good, not too bad. . . . I'm on Social Security and have my retirement, and I can live comfortably. Is that going to be enough? To be 40 years old and on

disability, especially knowing my occupational history, I don't know if that's going to be a long-term thing. Sometimes I feel like I should be doing more, and then my therapist has to remind me that I'm having a good run, but that I've got a chronic condition. I've had to come to a space of acceptance with that . . . , but I certainly won't be getting back into a career field.

The weight of the impact of TBI on today and tomorrow is a heavy load to carry. As a result, several veterans with TBI expressed a desire to live in the moment. For example, one veteran said, "I don't look towards the future. I look towards each day. New things to do. Future is to love and have fun with grandkids someday. Keep going strong even though things are happening the way they are." Although TBI presents many long-term difficulties and uncertainties for veterans, one strategy was to focus on the present and the aspects of life that could be managed.

Caregiver Experiences

Caregiver Challenges

The eight caregivers in the sample, who were mothers, female partners, and one male partner of a veteran with TBI, were forthcoming about the challenges of caring for their loved ones, as well as being a witness to their challenges. Some were new partners who were unfamiliar with military life, while others "had been training for this [their] whole life," having come from military families themselves. Regardless of how much experience the caregivers had, caregiving for a veteran with TBI and any associated comorbidities was an integral part of their day-to-day lives. This responsibility entailed being on call to run errands that the veteran could not handle, providing reminders to take prescriptions, and having patience beyond all normal expectations—all on top of quotidian tasks. Life was even more difficult if medical appointments were far away, which could easily happen when receiving care from a VA facility. One caregiver stated, "I can't go back to work, can't do something full-time, can't really leave him home alone."

Caregivers spoke about the VA Caregiver Support Program, but only two were successfully able to receive financial support; the others were not eligible for reasons that were unclear (and perceived to be unfair) to them. The Elizabeth Dole Foundation and WWP had provided some with additional support, such as paying for a nanny or housekeeper for six months after having children and providing the opportunity to take trips to meet with other military families in similar situations. Some of the caregivers expressed guilt for receiving support; as one noted, "I know the care that my husband needs, and then I see the people who are dealing with having an amputee husband or completely blind, and they're the people who really need to be in the programs. *They* need the extra respite." Another caregiver noted the stigma sometimes levied against them, remarking, "Some people in the community don't understand it either. I'm not home eating bonbons all day. I wish I did!"

Thus, the challenges for caregivers stretch from the workload to the emotional burden, as even relief can bring a cost.

Many caregivers detailed the necessity of strongly advocating on behalf of their partner to receive proper care. This took two forms: (1) pushing for the correct medical care in a complex and sometimes disjointed system and (2) fighting to ensure that health care costs were covered. Caregivers often gave accounts of going beyond what the health care system recommended. One wife added, "I'm a strong advocate of fighting for one's health care and doing one's own research. So much of the injury is unfixable, but all of the pharmaceuticals aren't touching it, so what else can we try?" When describing why they needed to advocate for their partners, caregivers mentioned the challenges of different systems interfacing to share information, the complicated nature of TBI, and the amount that is unknown about the condition. One caregiver cited the breaks in lines of communication across DoD and VA, noting, "Getting communication between military records and different care he had carried over to the VA system was hard, and then making sure it got put in correctly and getting them to actually look over past records. Everything was a total rehash!" Some caregivers said that repeating tests and consultations, at times, still did not lead to a clear treatment plan. Another caregiver echoed that VA and DoD do not "work well together at all." One caregiver explained that employees of VA sometimes looked at her and her husband suspiciously, thinking the couple was only interested in boosting his disability rating to receive greater financial compensation. She noted that she learned to push past this and encouraged other caregivers to do the same to get their veterans' needed health care. This experience also led her to worry about veterans who do not have such an advocate.

Part of the fight for appropriate health care includes ensuring that the expenses are covered. This can involve deciphering which party will cover health care costs. Submitting the necessary documentation felt invasive to one caregiver, who explained, "One thing that frosts me is that before they really help us, they want all of our financial records and tax records before they'll help us. WWP is one of them. They wanted me to fill out a huge pamphlet and wanted information on savings account balances." In this instance, the caregiver gave up on the process. Even after that step, the struggle to have the health care paid for, especially when it may be less conventional, can make it not worth the effort:

> A lot of these things actually do help him—massage therapy—but it's temporary relief. But the VA won't cover the care, or the few times that they do, it's such a difficult process to get reimbursed. . . . TRICARE doesn't cover it. The VA even through Choice doesn't cover it. It winds up being a lot of out-of-pocket expense. Then it was causing so much extra mental, physical, emotional stress that we said, "You know what? We're done. After three years, we're done. We'll come for maintenance visits but that's it." By doing that, quality of life has improved dramatically.

The bureaucracy and culture of the systems that oversee the payment of benefits can be so discouraging that veterans with TBI may not be receiving the health care and services they need, and caregivers are not guaranteed support for their own challenges.

Caregiver Concerns

Caregivers expressed concerns about long-term issues related to TBI and other health impacts for their children and partners. The caregivers have accepted that their veteran with TBI will face additional challenges later in life. They shared the concern that the "VA is not prepared, and the onus is going to be on the caregivers and spouses." As a result, some caregivers structure their life choices regarding employment, financial planning, children, and retirement to meet the long-term care needs. As one caregiver stated, "I think about long-term care. I don't want to stop living to just take care of him. I want to have enough resources to ensure that my quality of life is still there." Nevertheless, some caregivers and their partners face the uncertainty of the future with a sense of peace: "There's the possibility of future developments in the kind of care that she gets that could increase her level of freedom, but we're both very grateful for how effective the care that she receives is. We understand that no one knows what the future holds, but that is true for anyone." Although the caregivers were hopeful for advancements in care down the road, they stayed focused on the here and now. Parents also wonder what will happen to the child with TBI after the parents are no longer able to provide care or need care themselves. Our interviewees said that they have made plans for that future, such as turning over caregiving duties to a sibling of the wounded veteran. The mother of one veteran said, "My heartfelt request to my daughter is that she would direct his [the veteran's] care but not become a full-time caregiver. Her reply is that she would do everything she could, but her brother will not be institutionalized as long as she's alive." As a parent, the concern for the child's well-being is profound and not easily resolved. The challenges of being a caregiver today are real, and the long-term responsibilities impose additional worries.

Caregiver Family Impact

Having a family member with TBI affects families in many ways. In daily living, the caregiver often picks up the practical and emotional slack. Caregivers spoke about anticipating and accommodating the limitations of the veterans. In terms of emotional bandwidth, that can mean, "If there's something that's too much, we won't look at it." Thus, being aware of the effects of TBI and adjusting to it is a strategy that families employ to make life easier for the veteran. One mother explained that she, her husband, and her adult daughter (who lives at home) all take care of her son with TBI, and she described it as "this great little ballet." Unfortunately, some of the impacts can have a negative toll on families. Families can suffer the emotional consequences of a member with TBI who has trouble regulating him- or herself. One veteran said, "The people who suffer the consequences the most are the family. My 12-year-old son wasn't around when I got injured. Now he's starting to understand it on a different level rather than 'Daddy is being a jerk' and Daddy really doesn't want to be that way." It is asking a lot of a child to make sense of such behaviors even if he can begin to understand them over time. The downside, though, can lead to burnout for caregivers, especially when substance abuse is involved. Although a horrific opioid-related incident had occurred years prior, one wife's voice still shook as she described the details and the moment she told her husband that she was taking the kids and leaving. He eventually came to terms with his addiction, and they remained together. Thus, living with a family member with TBI is a delicate and shifting balance that requires patience, planning, and perseverance.

Caregiver Support

To cope with the challenges of tending to a family member with TBI, caregivers often seek both formal and informal means of support. As noted earlier, several (but not all) caregivers in our sample were able to secure support from VA or from service organizations, such as the Elizabeth Dole Foundation and WWP. The caregivers commonly relied on other family and friends for emotional and practical assistance. Having friends "who can read between the lines and say, 'You want to come spend the night or come over, have a glass of wine?'" helped sustain caregivers through the ups and downs. Caregivers also noted that they will call on friends and family for help when they cannot be present; one person cited the benefit of having others who can be around when the veteran is having seizures, because tending to the veteran in that situation requires skills and knowledge that not everyone possesses. Several caregivers also spoke about the strength they draw through their spirituality. One person said, "God has had me in basic training for being my son's advocate my entire life." It was clear to many caregivers that their religious grounding was instrumental to their ability to persevere through the challenges they faced.

Having a network of fellow caregivers can also be a great benefit. Peers have a special understanding of the experience and often share knowledge about useful resources. The network can become self-propagating. One wife described that "just knowing that there is a safety net with caregivers is helpful. I have connected more caregivers to resources than I have used. I love people and I'm happy when my house is full with others. It gives me joy to connect people." Another wife described a network of military wives that formed when a nonprofit organization provided them with a weekend of pampering while their veteran husbands were away on a weekend trip to the outdoors. Those caregivers subsequently formed an alumni Facebook group. On the other hand, some caregivers were looking for a support network but did not know where to find one. For example, one heard that VA offers caregiver support but did not know how it worked. Others were open to joining such a network of other caregivers but did not feel a great need to find such a group.

Suggestions for Improved Support

Both veterans and caregivers offered many suggestions for improved care and support. Many stated that they wanted more support groups for veterans. One wife of a veteran shared, "If WWP got a group of us together that have experiences with TBI and need help and are trying to get help, share their experiences in an open room, talking with each other, sharing symptoms—if you're together in a group of other veterans, you feel safe." Being a veteran and experiencing a TBI are both unique and challenging experiences, so several of those interviewed thought that increasing the chances to share with and support one another would be very valuable. The preference was for this to happen in person when possible. Similarly, another veteran suggested a mentorship program: "You're forced to have a battle buddy when you're in, but why not when you're out? Why not a mentor?" Several veterans expressed that they try to provide informal mentoring to others, so this seems to be an idea that would be well received. The veterans also mentioned trying to help other veterans navigate the VA system, but one suggested assigning specific case managers to the task:

> It really helps when they have the case managers to help get compensation. They should have more people helping the soldiers to point them in the right direction, to let them know what they have to do. For TBI, for instance, have a person who looks over your medical records and asks you the questions about what's going on with you, what are you experiencing. But don't wait so late! Do that when they first get back! The VA is not going to be as proactive.

As in other fields, case managers could provide comprehensive support for the clients to assist them in all aspects of their health care, including system navigation and basic health status. Along those lines, one veteran commented that VA needs to do a much better job of connecting veterans to disability evaluations. Perhaps a case manager could help with this too.

Several people wanted more programming for veterans in rural areas. One veteran offered this representative point: "There's a lot of folks who don't like cities, don't like being in the crowd, and they live in rural places, and there aren't enough resources in rural areas. That's VA and it's WWP." One veteran emphasized the importance of having programs in person, including in Montana (in more places than Helena), where a large concentration of veterans reside. Nevertheless, many wanted to see a greater use of telehealth, particularly for mental health treatment. Others thought that better capitalizing on technology, such as mobile devices with calendars or other memory aids, was an opportunity for growth and support. Related to these, one veteran wanted to see more cognitive classes to work on memory or other tasks, and these classes could be online too. Others spoke of the benefits from alternative treatments, such as receiving acupuncture, visiting a chiropractor, and taking some currently illicit drugs, so they wanted to see more of these alternatives offered and their costs reimbursed.

For caregivers, a common suggestion was to offer additional help across basic life tasks. Financial assistance was also mentioned by one wife of a veteran, who said with a laugh, "The wives need a wife! I hate to say money; it's not the solution, but it does allow for things like respite, a housekeeper, activities for the caregiver to get a massage or whatever. But I also don't think just throwing money at the problem is the solution." Finally, one caregiver wanted more guidance about aging for veterans with PTSD and TBI:

> There are enough veterans with PTSD and TBI that they can start to have some plans in place. Provide handouts for caregivers. If you notice XYZ, tell your doctor, here's what to

be prepared for. The VA can offer additional care for [occupational therapy], cognitive tests. A lot of people with PTSD have a hard time with focus. If the VA takes some of that on for our veterans, offer more than just physical therapy; [they] need to work on brain dexterity. It's a use it or lose it, your brain. If you have trauma with external factors, some of that can accelerate the aging process. If the VA were to get in front of that, if they were proactive instead of reactive, it would benefit them and the veterans they serve.

Because the challenges to the brain and aging are so big, the caregiver strongly expressed a desire for more information and direction. Although much is still not known about how TBI will affect veterans now and in the future, caregivers and veterans want to proactively do the work to help themselves. These suggestions were focused on capitalizing on the affected individuals' own motivations and resources to prepare themselves for the future.

Summary

The sample of veterans who volunteered to participate in an interview skewed toward those with moderate or severe TBI, which may explain why the majority of veterans in the sample reported enduring serious challenges. Complications in treating their TBI began right from the combat zone, where some then–service members were reluctant or unable to seek care for a TBI. As a result, many reported sustaining several TBIs before suffering one definitive blow that was accompanied by other physical injuries. Receiving a diagnosis and timely treatment was hardly straightforward, and many veterans had to seek treatment for many years in several different locations with varying degrees of care. Veterans' search for care and perceived success with treatment were further complicated by comorbid conditions, especially PTSD, migraines, and cognitive challenges, which were pervasive across this sample of veterans.

The cognitive challenges that many veterans expressed difficulty with included remembering what to get from the grocery store and following a conversation. Such challenges have taken a major toll on veterans' identities, their ability to seek employment and educational opportunities, their romantic relationships, and the well-being of their families, which was confirmed by their caregivers. Several veterans have coped with these challenges through service, particularly service to other veterans.

It is important to note that this qualitative analysis focused on veterans who were injured several years prior to the interview, and both basic science and clinical research on TBI, as well as delivery of health services, have made important strides in recent years. These experiences may not reflect those of veterans who were treated more recently or those who did not volunteer to participate in an interview. That being said, clinicians and researchers cannot lose sight of the needs of the aging veterans who did not have access to newer treatments and may therefore be facing additional challenges and service needs.

Looking to the future, veterans in this sample were concerned about accelerated aging and early-onset dementia. They were looking for answers and ways to prepare, and some suggested that access to portable or wearable technologies may help relieve the cognitive burden they are facing. The veterans were proactively working through their reported limitations and leveraging their resources to establish a new normal.

Treatments and Interventions to Address Long-Term Outcomes for Veterans with Traumatic Brain Injury

In this chapter, we document the current research (up to July 2021) on treatment approaches for long-term outcomes following TBI and present an evidence map to visually display the current state of research on TBI treatment, including where the evidence is robust and where it is sparse. To guide the evidence map, we asked, *Which TBI treatment approaches have been collectively and rigorously evaluated in systematic reviews?*

Approach to the Umbrella Review of Traumatic Brain Injury Treatments and Interventions

We began the literature review by developing search terms for four databases that are widely used to index relevant research: PubMed, PsycInfo, Web of Science, and PROSPERO (Appendix C). Our goal was to identify English-language, peer-reviewed literature on the effectiveness of interventions to address long-term outcomes associated with TBI. We identified systematic reviews and meta-analyses of interventions that targeted post-acute interventions for long-term outcomes in adult TBI populations. TBI interventions are often tested across acute and chronic settings; in adults, children, and adolescents; and within other disease states (e.g., stroke). Therefore, we included systematic reviews in which at least 50 percent of the included studies examined chronic intervention implementation, adults, and TBI-specific diagnosis.

Eligibility Criteria

To operationalize the review question, study eligibility criteria were defined using the following PICOTSS (population, intervention, comparators, outcomes, timing, setting, and study design) framework:

- *Population:* We included systematic reviews involving adults with a TBI of any severity. Systematic reviews that included a mix of studies on adults with those on children or adolescents were included only if the majority of studies in the review involved adults.

- *Intervention:* We included systematic reviews of interventions to treat symptoms and clinical sequelae of TBI. These studies included peer-to-peer interventions, workplace-organized interventions, and adjuvant wellness interventions, among others. We excluded interventions during the acute phase of treatment—for example, neurosurgery.
- *Comparators:* Studies were not restricted by comparator.
- *Outcomes:* We included systematic reviews that broadly assessed long-term outcomes associated with TBI in the following categories: cognitive, psychological, functional, physical, social, occupational, and PCS.
- *Timing:* We did not place any restrictions related to publication year, the length of the intervention, or the length of the follow-up period.
- *Setting:* We included systematic reviews in any treatment setting, although many studies in the inpatient setting were excluded because they described interventions provided during the acute phase of care.
- *Study design:* We included systematic reviews of quantitative human subjects studies assessing the effects of interventions on long-term outcomes among people with TBI. We did not exclude studies based on study design (e.g., randomized control trial, pre or post, quasi-experimental). We excluded scoping reviews and narrative syntheses.
- *Other limiters:* We restricted the review to English-language publications so that we could provide a transparent and readily available resource catalog of interventions. We excluded dissertations and all studies reported in abbreviated formats (e.g., conference abstracts, letters to the editor).

Data Extraction

We created a data extraction form that included detailed instructions and decision rules for reviewers so that we could maintain a standardized data-collection process. To ensure consistency of interpretation of all fields on the form, reviewers pilot-tested a draft version of the form on a few studies for which results were clearly reported. We iteratively modified and tested the form with randomly selected samples of eligible studies until arriving at the final version. One reviewer extracted data from included studies, and a second reviewer checked the data for accuracy. We resolved any discrepancies through discussion among the review team.

The data extraction form focused on key information needed to display the evidence in an evidence map and provide a brief evidence table. First, we categorized participants into three groups: veterans, athletes, and the general adult population (or a combination thereof). Second, we characterized the type of intervention (e.g., pharmacotherapy, psychotherapy) and the type of outcome (e.g., cognitive, psychological). We did not systematically perform a critical appraisal of each study included in the systematic reviews.

Synthesis

To summarize evidence within each study, we broadly categorized the interventions and the outcomes of the interventions in terms of effectiveness according to the authors' summary. To synthesize evidence across studies, we created an evidence map of the effectiveness of interventions for specific outcomes associated with TBI. (The evidence map is presented later in this chapter.) To synthesize evidence across studies, we incorporated the following dimensions into the evidence map:

- The **y-axis** depicts the types of interventions that were tested (pharmacotherapy, psychotherapy, physical rehabilitation, occupational rehabilitation, cognitive rehabilitation, behavioral rehabilitation, virtual care, care coordination, physical exercise, brain stimulation, hyperbaric oxygen therapy, complementary and alternative medicine).
- The **x-axis** depicts the categories of long-term outcomes assessed in the systematic reviews (cognitive, psychological, functional, physical, social, occupational, PCS).
- The **shape** of the icons represents the population in which the interventions were tested (veterans, athletes, general adult population, or a combination thereof).
- The **color** of the icons represents the effectiveness of the intervention in the respective systematic review (yes, no, mixed, unclear).
- The **size** of the icons represents the number of studies that assessed the intervention on the long-term outcome.

We identified several categories of long-term outcomes with varying corresponding interventions. We made operational decisions to categorize interventions and long-term outcomes, and those categories are outlined in Table 5.1 with examples.

Included Studies

Our initial combined search yielded 1,330 articles. We then conducted one round of abstract review and two rounds of full-text review and abstraction. The evidence map includes 2,847 publications from 165 systematic reviews that resulted in 327 studies that assessed the intervention on the long-term outcome. Figure 5.1 is a flow diagram of included and excluded systematic reviews, and Figure 5.2 presents the evidence map.

TABLE 5.1

Categories and Examples of Interventions and Long-Term Outcomes

Category	Examples
Interventions (y-axis)	
Pharmacotherapy	Pharmacotherapy for physical or psychological symptoms
Psychotherapy	Cognitive behavioral therapy
Physical rehabilitation	Physical therapy, speech or language therapy, oculomotor therapy
Occupational rehabilitation	Occupational therapy, vocation-based rehabilitation, sensory stimulation
Cognitive rehabilitation	Neurocognitive rehabilitation, narrative discourse
Behavioral rehabilitation	Comprehensive rehabilitation, education, rest, peer mentoring and support, community-based intervention
Virtual care	Virtual reality, telehealth, smartphone-based interventions
Care coordination	Case management, multidisciplinary rehabilitation
Physical exercise	Aerobic exercise
Brain stimulation	Transcranial magnetic stimulation
Hyperbaric oxygen therapy	
Complementary and alternative medicine	Acupuncture, light therapy
Long-Term Outcomes (x-axis)	
Cognitive	Attention, memory, executive function
Psychological	Depression, anxiety, PTSD, substance misuse, aggression
Functional	Activities of daily living, balance, gait
Physical	Physical or physiological symptoms, sleep, cardiorespiratory symptoms, seizure, headache, vision, speech
Social	Community integration, social engagement, quality of life
Occupational	Return to work, school, or service; financial health
PCS	

FIGURE 5.1

Flow Diagram of Included and Excluded Studies on Treatments and Interventions to Address Long-Term Outcomes Following Traumatic Brain Injury

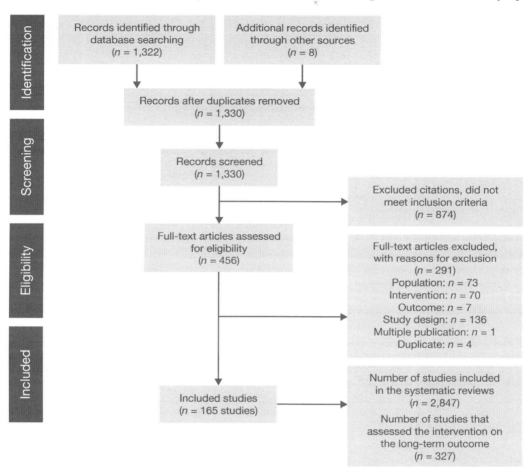

FIGURE 5.2

Evidence Map of Interventions and Long-Term Outcomes for Traumatic Brain Injury

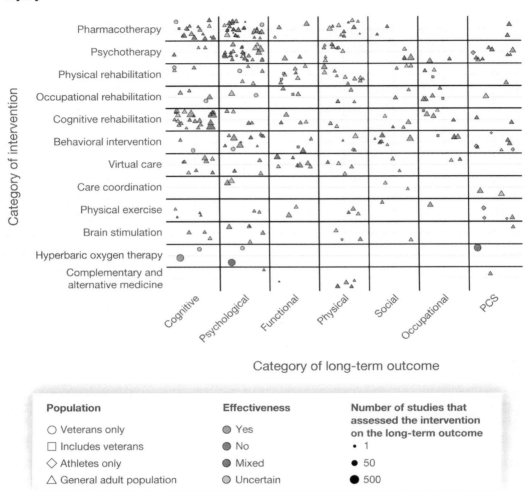

Strength of Evidence for Interventions, by Outcome Type

Findings were mixed for the effect of heterogeneous interventions on clinically meaningful outcomes. In reporting findings, we classify them into four categories: (1) there was evidence that an intervention was effective on a category of outcomes; (2) there was evidence that an intervention was not associated with a category of outcomes (i.e., the review demonstrated no effect); (3) the findings within a single review were mixed, containing evidence for and against an intervention being effective for an outcome category; and (4) the authors of the systematic review concluded that the findings were uncertain or inconclusive or that the evidence was too weak to draw a conclusion. This final category often co-occurred in systematic reviews that indicated high potential for bias, low-quality evidence, or both. In this section, we detail the types of interventions tested against the seven categories of outcomes and the systematic reviews' stated effectiveness of those interventions in veteran, athlete, general adult, or mixed populations. Unless otherwise indicated, results are for the general adult population.

Cognitive

Most interventions for cognitive outcomes were pharmacotherapy, cognitive rehabilitation, or virtual care. Cognitive rehabilitation and virtual care had the most evidence for effectiveness for improving cognitive outcomes, and a small number of systematic reviews demonstrated the effectiveness of brain stimulation interventions. Little evidence came from veteran-only populations or populations that included veterans.

Seventeen systematic reviews assessed the effects of pharmacotherapy on cognition. Four of these demonstrated effectiveness (Chien et al., 2019; Meshkini, Meshkini, and Sadeghi-Bazargani, 2017; Mohamed et al., 2021; Szarka et al., 2021), and two presented evidence that pharmacotherapy was not effective for improving cognitive outcomes (Frenette et al., 2012; Lyons and Blackshaw, 2018); only one of these reviews included veterans (Lyons and Blackshaw, 2018). Seven systematic reviews presented mixed findings for the effect of pharmacotherapy on cognition (Anghinah et al., 2018; Bengtsson and Godbolt, 2016; Dougall, Poole, and Agrawal, 2015; Iaccarino et al., 2020; Sivan et al., 2010; Wheaton, Mathias, and Vink, 2011; Writer and Schillerstrom, 2009), and four systematic reviews concluded that overall findings were uncertain or that there was insufficient evidence (Ballesteros et al., 2008; Hicks et al., 2018; Sami and Faruqui, 2015; Wilson et al., 2016), one of which focused exclusively on veterans (Wilson et al., 2016). Three systematic reviews assessed the effect of psychotherapy on cognitive outcomes, again to varying effect: one positive (Mahan, Rous, and Adlam, 2017), one with mixed findings (Snell et al., 2009), and one that had uncertain conclusions (Bergersen et al., 2017).

Likewise, three systematic reviews assessed the effects of physical rehabilitation on cognition, and one demonstrated positive effects in the general adult population (Fritz, Cheek, and Nichols-Larsen, 2015). Of the other two systematic reviews, one exclusively examined populations of veterans (Wilson et al., 2016), and one drew uncertain conclusions (Brassel et al., 2021). Four systematic reviews assessed the effects of occupational rehabilitation interventions on cognition. The three systematic reviews examining the general adult population demonstrated effectiveness (Park, Maitra, and Martinez, 2015; Pinto et al., 2020; Radomski et al., 2016), but the one that exclusively included populations of veterans was uncertain in its conclusions (Wilson et al., 2016). Twenty-three systematic reviews, all examining the general adult population, assessed the effect of cognitive rehabilitation on cognitive outcomes. Fourteen of those reviews demonstrated effectiveness (Bogdanova et al., 2016; Cicerone et al., 2005; Cicerone et al., 2011; Elliott and Parente, 2014; Fritz, Cheek, and Nichols-Larsen, 2015; Hallock et al., 2016; Kennedy et al., 2008; Lambez and Vakil, 2021; Little, Byrne, and Coetzer, 2021; O'Neil-Pirozzi, Kennedy, and Sohlberg, 2016; Park, Maitra, and Martinez,

2015; Radomski et al., 2016; Rodríguez-Rajo et al., 2018; Rohling et al., 2009), and two demonstrated no effect (Chung et al., 2013; Virk et al., 2015). Additionally, three reviews had mixed findings (Cicerone et al., 2019; Roitsch et al., 2019; Steel, Elbourn, and Togher, 2021), and four characterized the evidence as uncertain (Ali, Viczko, and Smart, 2020; Brassel et al., 2021; Geraldo et al., 2018; Schrijnemaekers et al., 2014). Two systematic reviews assessed the effect of behavioral rehabilitation on cognitive outcomes, demonstrating effectiveness in the general adult population (Little, Byrne, and Coetzer, 2021) and uncertain conclusions in populations restricted to veterans (Wilson et al., 2016).

Eight studies assessed the effectiveness of virtual care in the general adult population. Five of the reviews demonstrated positive effects (Alashram et al., 2019; Betts et al., 2018; Bogdanova et al., 2016; Leopold et al., 2015; Voinescu, Sui, and Fraser, 2021), one found mixed effects (Manivannan et al., 2019), and two drew uncertain conclusions (Brassel et al., 2021; Buhagiar et al., 2020). Physical exercise was tested for cognitive effects in four systematic reviews. Two studies demonstrated no effect (McDonnell, Smith, and Mackintosh, 2011; Sharma et al., 2020), one demonstrated mixed effects (Vanderbeken and Kerckhofs, 2017), and one drew uncertain conclusions (Morris et al., 2016). Three systematic reviews assessed the effect of brain stimulation on cognition; two reviews showed positive effectiveness (Ahorsu, Adjaottor, and Lam, 2021; Dhaliwal, Meek, and Modirrousta, 2015), and one drew uncertain conclusions (Buhagiar et al., 2020). Two studies tested the effect of hyperbaric oxygen therapy on cognition in populations restricted to veterans. One demonstrated effectiveness (Hart et al., 2019), and one drew uncertain conclusions (Wilson et al., 2016).

Psychological

Most systematic reviews of psychological outcomes assessed pharmacotherapy and psychotherapy interventions. Evidence was strongest for psychotherapy and, to a lesser extent, physical exercise and brain stimulation. Some systematic reviews of psychotherapy included populations restricted to veterans.

Twenty-nine systematic reviews assessed the effectiveness of pharmacotherapy on psychological outcomes. Eight of these reviews demonstrated positive effects (Beedham et al., 2020; Fann, Hart, and Schomer, 2009; Hicks et al., 2019; Hicks et al., 2020; Meshkini, Meshkini, and Sadeghi-Bazargani, 2017; Peppel, Ribbers, and Heijenbrok-Kal, 2020; Sami and Faruqui, 2015; Szarka et al., 2021). Conversely, seven systematic reviews demonstrated no effect of pharmacotherapy on psychological outcomes (Ackland et al., 2019; Cheng et al., 2021; Gao et al., 2019; Kreitzer et al., 2019; Paraschakis and Katsanos, 2017; Reyes, Espiritu, and Anlacan, 2019; Salter et al., 2016), and one of those reviews examined populations restricted to veterans (Ackland et al., 2019). Furthermore, seven systematic reviews presented mixed results (Barker-Collo, Starkey, and Theadom, 2013; Iaccarino et al., 2020; Jin and Schachar, 2004; Maksimowski and Tampi, 2016; Narapareddy et al., 2020; Rahmani et al., 2021; Wheaton, Mathias, and Vink, 2011). Seven additional systematic reviews arrived at uncertain conclusions about the effect of pharmacotherapy on psychological outcomes (Carlson et al., 2009; Clay et al., 2019; Hicks et al., 2021; Matarazzo et al., 2013; Sami and Faruqui, 2015; Slowinski,

Coetzer, and Byrne, 2019; Wilson et al., 2016), and three of those focused exclusively on veterans (Hicks et al., 2021; Matarazzo et al., 2013; Wilson et al., 2016).

Twenty-four systematic reviews of psychotherapy demonstrated slightly more evidence of effectiveness, though still mixed effects, on psychological outcomes. Half ($n = 12$) demonstrated the effectiveness of psychotherapy for improving psychological outcomes, all in the general adult population (Ackland et al., 2019; Beedham et al., 2020; Cattelani, Zettin, and Zoccolotti, 2010; Chung and Khan, 2013; Fann, Hart, and Schomer, 2009; Iruthayarajah et al., 2018; Lane-Brown and Tate, 2009b; Möller, Lexell, and Wilbe Ramsay, 2021; Peppel, Ribbers, and Heijenbrok-Kal, 2020; Soo and Tate, 2007; Swedish Agency for Health Technology Assessment and Assessment of Social Services, 2019; Thomas et al., 2017). Three systematic reviews found no effectiveness of psychotherapy for psychological outcomes (Cheng et al., 2021; Gertler, Tate, and Cameron, 2015; Liu, Zeng, and Duan, 2018). Six systematic reviews, including one that studied (but was not limited to) veteran populations (Mikolić et al., 2019), demonstrated mixed findings (Barker-Collo, Starkey, and Theadom, 2013; Mueller et al., 2018; Ownsworth and Haslam, 2016; Snell et al., 2009; Wiart et al., 2016), and three additional systematic reviews arrived at uncertain conclusions (Argyriou et al., 2021; Carlson et al., 2009; Matarazzo et al., 2013).

The effect of physical rehabilitation on psychological outcomes was assessed in five systematic reviews. Two found positive associations (Möller, Lexell, and Wilbe Ramsay, 2021; Thomas et al., 2017), and three found uncertain conclusions (Argyriou et al., 2021; Brassel et al., 2021; Wilson et al., 2016). The only systematic review that included the effect of physical rehabilitation on psychological outcomes in a population exclusively composed of veterans concluded that findings were uncertain (Wilson et al., 2016). Occupational rehabilitation for psychological outcomes was tested in two systematic reviews, both of which reached uncertain conclusions (Swedish Agency for Health Technology Assessment and Assessment of Social Services, 2019; Wilson et al., 2016); one examined veteran populations only (Wilson et al., 2016). Two systematic reviews found cognitive rehabilitation to be effective (Chung and Khan, 2013; Little, Byrne, and Coetzer, 2021), one had mixed findings (Ownsworth and Haslam, 2016), and one had uncertain conclusions (Brassel et al., 2021). Behavioral rehabilitation was assessed for psychological outcomes in 11 systematic reviews, six of which demonstrated a positive effect (Cattelani, Zettin, and Zoccolotti, 2010; Little, Byrne, and Coetzer, 2021; Möller, Lexell, and Wilbe Ramsay, 2021; Morris, Fletcher-Smith, and Radford, 2017; Wobma et al., 2016; Ylvisaker et al., 2007) and two of which demonstrated mixed effects (Mueller et al., 2018; Ownsworth and Haslam, 2016). Of the three systematic reviews that stated uncertain effects of behavioral interventions on psychological outcomes (Bahraini et al., 2013; Bogner and Corrigan, 2013; Wilson et al., 2016), one assessed populations restricted to veterans (Wilson et al., 2016).

Three systematic reviews assessed the effectiveness of virtual care for psychological outcomes. One demonstrated effectiveness (Thomas et al., 2017), one had mixed findings (Ownsworth et al., 2018), and one arrived at uncertain conclusions (Brassel et al., 2021). Domains of care coordination were assessed to positive and uncertain effect on varied psychological outcomes in one review (Swedish Agency for Health Technology Assessment and Assessment of Social Services, 2019). Physical exercise was effective for improving psychological outcomes in two systematic reviews (Hassett, Moseley, and Harmer, 2017; Perry, Coetzer, and Saville, 2020). Likewise, brain stimulation was effective in three of five reviews (Beedham et al., 2020; Dhaliwal, Meek, and Modirrousta, 2015; Narapareddy et al., 2020); of the other two, one demonstrated no effectiveness (Lane-Brown and Tate, 2009a), and one demonstrated uncertain conclusions (Argyriou et al., 2021). Of two systematic reviews that assessed psychological outcomes from hyperbaric oxygen therapy, one found it to be not effective (Hart et al., 2019), and the other had uncertain conclusions (Wilson et al., 2016). One study of complementary and alternative medicine demonstrated a positive effect on psychological outcomes (Srisurapanont et al., 2021).

Functional

Systematic reviews of functional outcomes most frequently assessed physical rehabilitation and virtual care. Evidence of the effectiveness for improving functional outcomes was mixed across intervention types but had the most proportionally positive associations in a small number of systematic reviews of occupational rehabilitation. None exclusively included populations of veterans.

Two of the three systematic reviews of functional outcomes and pharmacotherapy interventions demonstrated effectiveness (Marshall et al., 2007; Szarka et al., 2021); one showed uncertain conclusions (Sami and Faruqui, 2015). Likewise, of the two systematic reviews of functional outcomes that focused on psychotherapy interventions, one demonstrated a positive effect (Marshall et al., 2007) and one mixed effectiveness (Snell et al., 2009).

Nine systematic reviews assessed the effect of physical rehabilitation on functional outcomes. Three of these reviews demonstrated effectiveness (Cullen et al., 2007; Hellweg and Johannes, 2008; Renzenbrink et al., 2012), including one that included populations of veterans (Cullen et al., 2007); one review did not demonstrate effectiveness (Alashram et al., 2020), and five were uncertain (Bland, Zampieri, and Damiano, 2011; Brassel et al., 2021; Lannin and McCluskey, 2008; Murray, Meldrum, and Lennon, 2017; Postol et al., 2019), one of which included populations of veterans (Murray, Meldrum, and Lennon, 2017). Occupational rehabilitation was found to be effective in three systematic reviews (Cullen et al., 2007; Pinto et al., 2020; Powell, Rich, and Wise, 2016), one of which included populations of veterans (Cullen et al., 2007). The effect of cognitive rehabilitation was assessed in four systematic reviews: Two found that it was effective (Carney et al., 1999; Hallock et al., 2016), one did not demonstrate effectiveness (Chung et al., 2013), and one reached uncertain conclusions (Brassel et al., 2021). Of the three reviews examining behavioral interventions for functional outcomes, two had positive findings (Cullen et al., 2007; Tate, Wakim, and Genders, 2014), one of which examined populations of veterans (Cullen et al., 2007), and one had mixed results (McCabe et al., 2007).

Virtual care was tested in seven systematic reviews that assessed functional outcomes, all in the general adult population. Two demonstrated effectiveness (Leopold et al., 2015;

Voinescu, Sui, and Fraser, 2021), one did not (Alashram et al., 2020), two had mixed findings (Ownsworth et al., 2018; Sigmundsdottir, Longley, and Tate, 2016), and two drew uncertain conclusions (Brassel et al., 2021; Postol et al., 2019). Physical exercise was assessed for its effect on functional outcomes in two systematic reviews examining the general adult population. In one, physical exercise was found to be effective (Marshall et al., 2007), and in the other, findings led to uncertain conclusions (Postol et al., 2019). Complementary and alternative medicine was found to be effective for improving functional outcomes in one systematic review of studies of the general adult population (Davidson et al., 2011).

Physical

Most interventions for physical outcomes were pharmacotherapy, psychotherapy, or physical rehabilitation. Although there was positive evidence for multiple types of interventions, systematic reviews of physical outcomes included a high number of uncertain conclusions. All but one analysis of physical outcomes were conducted in the general adult population.

Pharmacotherapy was assessed for its effect on physical outcomes in 11 systematic reviews; in none was it found to be effective. One systematic review demonstrated no effect of pharmacotherapy on physical outcomes (Wilson et al., 2018), and the findings in the other ten reviews were either mixed (Borghol et al., 2018; Iaccarino et al., 2020; Pilon, Frankenmolen, and Bertens, 2021; Sheng et al., 2013) or uncertain (Barlow et al., 2019; Cantor et al., 2014; Lew et al., 2006; Synnot et al., 2017; Watanabe et al., 2012; Zhao et al., 2018). Psychotherapy effectively improved physical outcomes in three studies (Bogdanov, Naismith, and Lah, 2017; Lowe et al., 2020; Pilon, Frankenmolen, and Bertens, 2021), with mixed results in another (Snell et al., 2009); conclusions were uncertain in five systematic reviews (Argyriou et al., 2021; Bergersen et al., 2017; Cantor et al., 2014; Lew et al., 2006; Sullivan et al., 2018).

The effects of physical rehabilitation on physical outcomes were assessed in ten systematic reviews. The intervention type was found to be effective in four reviews (Fritz, Cheek, and Nichols-Larsen, 2015; Kinne et al., 2018; Watabe et al., 2019; Yu et al., 2017) and findings were uncertain in six (Argyriou et al., 2021; Brassel et al., 2021; Cheever et al., 2021; Lew et al., 2006; Postol et al., 2019; Synnot et al., 2017). Occupational rehabilitation had positive (Chang, Baxter, and Rissky, 2016), mixed (Berger et al., 2016), and uncertain (Synnot et al., 2017) findings in three studies that examined physical outcomes. Cognitive rehabilitation was found to be effective (Fritz, Cheek, and Nichols-Larsen, 2015) and to have uncertain effectiveness (Brassel et al., 2021) in two studies that assessed that intervention's association with physical outcomes. Physical outcomes were assessed in four systematic reviews of behavioral rehabilitation: Two reviews found the intervention to be effective (Bogdanov, Naismith, and Lah, 2017; Wobma et al., 2016), and two had uncertain conclusions (Minen, Jinich, and Vallespir Ellett, 2019; Watanabe et al., 2012).

The effect of virtual care on physical outcomes was assessed in four studies. In one, it was deemed effective (Chang, Baxter, and Rissky, 2016); in another, findings were mixed (Ownsworth et al., 2018); and in two others, the conclusions were uncertain (Brassel et al., 2021; Postol et al., 2019). Physical exercise was effective at improving physical outcomes in one systematic review (Lowe et al., 2020), showed mixed effect in another (Hassett, Moseley, and Harmer, 2017), and drew uncertain conclusions in a third (Postol et al., 2019). Brain stimulation effectively improved physical outcomes in one systematic review (Dhaliwal, Meek, and Modirrousta, 2015) and had uncertain conclusions in two studies (Argyriou et al., 2021; O'Neil et al., 2020), including one exclusively composed of veterans (O'Neil et al., 2020). Complementary and alternative medicine was effective at improving physical outcomes in three systematic reviews (Lowe et al., 2020; Srisurapanont et al., 2021; Xu et al., 2017), demonstrated mixed findings in one (Pilon, Frankenmolen, and Bertens, 2021), and drew uncertain conclusions in one (Cantor et al., 2014).

Social

Behavioral interventions were disproportionately tested for their effectiveness in social outcomes. There was positive and some mixed evidence for behavioral interventions, as well as positive evidence from a small number of systematic reviews that assessed the effects of occupational rehabilitation. All assessments of social outcomes were in conducted in the general adult population.

Pharmacotherapy effects were mixed for social outcomes, including one systematic review that demonstrated no effect (Reyes, Espiritu, and Anlacan, 2019) and one showing mixed effectiveness (Iaccarino et al., 2020). Psychotherapy improved social outcomes in two studies (Cattelani, Zettin, and Zoccolotti, 2010; Möller, Lexell, and Wilbe Ramsay, 2021), was of mixed effectiveness in one study (Snell et al., 2009), and was uncertain in one (Argyriou et al., 2021).

Physical rehabilitation was associated with improvements in social outcomes in one systematic review (Möller, Lexell, and Wilbe Ramsay, 2021) and uncertain effects in two others (Argyriou et al., 2021; Brassel et al., 2021). Occupational rehabilitation was found to be effective for social outcomes in two systematic reviews (Kim and Colantonio, 2010; Powell, Rich, and Wise, 2016). Cognitive rehabilitation was found to be effective in two systematic reviews (Carney et al., 1999; Rodríguez-Rajo et al., 2018), showed mixed effectiveness in one (Steel, Elbourn, and Togher, 2021), and drew uncertain conclusions in one (Brassel et al., 2021). Behavioral interventions for social outcomes were generally effective: Four systematic reviews demonstrated effectiveness (Cattelani, Zettin, and Zoccolotti, 2010; Finch et al., 2016; Möller, Lexell, and Wilbe Ramsay, 2021; Wobma et al., 2016), two demonstrated mixed effectiveness (McCabe et al., 2007; Morris, Fletcher-Smith, and Radford, 2017), and one had uncertain conclusions (Paice, Aleligay, and Checklin, 2020). Virtual care was effective in one systematic review for social outcomes (Betts et al., 2018), and a second review determined that conclusions were uncertain (Brassel et al., 2021). Care coordination showed uncertain conclusions for social outcomes in two systematic reviews (Brasure et al., 2013; Lannin et al., 2014); physical exercise was effective in one review (O'Carroll et al., 2020); and brain stimulation drew uncertain conclusions in one review (Argyriou et al., 2021).

Occupational

Systematic reviews most frequently examined the effects of occupational rehabilitation and cognitive rehabilitation for occupational outcomes. There was positive evidence for occupational rehabilitation, including in a small number of samples that included veterans. In small numbers of systematic reviews, there was also evidence of the effectiveness of behavioral interventions. None of those exclusively included veterans.

Psychotherapy was found to be effective for occupational outcomes in one systematic review (Wheeler, Acord-Vira, and Davis, 2016) and not effective in another (Thomas et al., 2017). Physical rehabilitation was assessed in three systematic reviews: It was effective in one review that included veterans (Cullen et al., 2007); when examining the general adult population, one systematic review indicated that physical rehabilitation was not effective (Thomas et al., 2017), and another determined that conclusions were uncertain (Brassel et al., 2021). Occupational rehabilitation effectively improved occupational outcomes in five systematic reviews (Cullen et al., 2007; Donker-Cools et al., 2016; Fadyl and McPherson, 2009; Radomski et al., 2016; Wheeler, Acord-Vira, and Davis, 2016). Cognitive rehabilitation was effective for improving occupational outcomes in two systematic reviews (Carney et al., 1999; Radomski et al., 2016), was not effective in one review (Chung et al., 2013), was of mixed effectiveness in one review that included populations of veterans (Kumar et al., 2017), and drew uncertain conclusions in a fifth systematic review (Brassel et al., 2021). Three behavioral interventions assessed occupational outcomes: Two demonstrated effectiveness (Cullen et al., 2007; Wheeler, Acord-Vira, and Davis, 2016), including one that included populations of veterans (Cullen et al., 2007), and one showed mixed effectiveness (McCabe et al., 2007). Virtual care of occupational outcomes was not effective in one systematic review (Thomas et al., 2017) and drew uncertain conclusions in a second (Brassel et al., 2021). Physical exercise was effective for improving occupational outcomes in one systematic review (Wheeler, Acord-Vira, and Davis, 2016).

Post-Concussion Syndrome

Psychotherapy and behavioral interventions were most frequently assessed for improving PCS outcomes. There was positive and mixed evidence for psychotherapy, as well as positive evidence for physical exercise, mostly from studies of athletes. Only one systematic review included veterans: a systematic review demonstrating no evidence for the effectiveness of hyperbaric oxygen therapy for PCS in populations restricted to veterans (Hart et al., 2019).

Two systematic reviews, one demonstrating no effectiveness (Arbabi et al., 2020) and one with mixed results (Comper et al., 2005), tested pharmacotherapy for PCS. More studies assessed psychotherapy for PCS. Three indicated that psychotherapy was effective for treating PCS (Arbabi et al., 2020; Makdissi et al., 2017; Swedish Agency for Health Technology Assessment and Assessment of Social Services, 2019), and six indicated mixed effectiveness (Al Sayegh, Sandford, and Carson, 2010; Chen et al., 2020; Chong, 2008; Nygren-de Boussard et al., 2014; Sullivan et al., 2020; Teo et al., 2020).

Physical rehabilitation was found to be effective for PCS in one systematic review (Arbabi et al., 2020), and occupational therapy had uncertain conclusions in one (Swedish Agency for Health Technology Assessment and Assessment of Social Services, 2019). Cognitive rehabilitation had mixed findings in two systematic reviews that assessed PCS (Comper et al., 2005; Teo et al., 2020). Three systematic reviews of behavioral rehabilitation among athletes found the intervention to be effective for reducing symptoms of PCS (Makdissi et al., 2017; Sawyer, Vesci, and McLeod, 2016; Schneider et al., 2013), one review examining the general adult population found no effectiveness (Arbabi et al., 2020), two found mixed effectiveness (Comper et al., 2005; Nygren-de Boussard et al., 2014), and one had uncertain conclusions (Minen, Jinich, and Vallespir Ellett, 2019). One systematic review provided two analyses of the effect of care coordination on PCS; effectiveness was positive for coordinated brain injury rehabilitation that included cognitive behavioral therapy, and the review concluded that effectiveness remained uncertain for multifaceted rehabilitation in more-severe injuries (Swedish Agency for Health Technology Assessment and Assessment of Social Services, 2019). Physical exercise was effective for improving PCS in three systematic reviews examining athletes only (Makdissi et al., 2017; Sawyer, Vesci, and McLeod, 2016; Schneider et al., 2013) and one systematic review examining the general adult population (Carter, Pauhl, and Christie, 2021). Brain stimulation was effective for PCS in one systematic review that looked at the general adult population (Mollica et al., 2021). Hyperbaric oxygen therapy was not effective in a systematic review that focused exclusively on veterans (Hart et al., 2019). One systematic review of the effects of complementary and alternative medicine on PCS found that it was effective in the general adult population (Acabchuk et al., 2021).

Discussion

The systematic reviews that we identified assessed diverse types of interventions, including pharmaco- and psychotherapy, various types of rehabilitation, brain stimulation, hyperbaric oxygen therapy, and complementary and alternative medicine. They likewise evaluated outcomes across multiple domains, such as cognitive, psychological, physical, and social outcomes. Overall, the strongest evidence supported that cognitive rehabilitation was effective for cognitive outcomes, psychotherapy was effective for psychological outcomes, behavioral interventions were effective for social outcomes, occupational rehabilitation was effective for occupational outcomes, and psychotherapy and behavioral interventions were effective for PCS. By comparison, findings on interventions for functional and physical outcomes were mixed. Authors of systematic reviews routinely emphasized the lack of high-quality evidence and the need for additional research with a low risk of bias, and the authors often were unwilling or unable to draw conclusions about an intervention's effectiveness. Understanding effective interventions for people living with long-term effects of TBI requires more research and higher-quality study designs.

Even for interventions that had higher-quality evidence for their effectiveness, that evidence overwhelmingly came from the general adult population rather than veterans. Veterans have experiences and etiologies of TBI that differ significantly enough from the general adult population that interventions may be disproportionately more or less effective among veterans. The differences may be due to etiology, population characteristics at baseline (including age and frailty), and physical and psychological comorbidity (e.g., physical trauma, baseline chronic conditions, PTSD). Even beyond veteran-specific concerns, many studies of interventions and long-term outcomes in TBI included broader acute brain injury diagnoses, which largely includes stroke. Although there are clinical population-based reasons for including TBI with other neurological conditions, it remains unclear whether interventions are equally effective across these populations. Likewise, many systematic reviews included a subset of studies or study populations that included children and adolescents, who may require significant developmental and rehabilitative differences in TBI treatments compared with even the general adult population. For these population-based reasons, it will be important for future work to include robust analyses and subanalyses of TBI-specific interventions in veteran populations when evaluating intervention outcomes with valid measurement tools (Polinder et al., 2015; Winkens et al., 2011).

Although stand-alone caregiver interventions and outcomes were beyond the scope of this review, the broader literature acknowledges that family caregivers who are involved in TBI recovery are essential for engagement with patients and bear large burdens that warrant robust intervention in their own right. That is, caregivers who support recovery for those with TBI also need practical, educational, and psychological support. Systematic reviews (not included in this study) have started to focus on or incorporate caregivers into interventions (Baker et al., 2017; Shepherd-Banigan, McDuffie, et al., 2018; Shepherd-Banigan, Shapiro, et al., 2018). Likewise, systematic reviews are increasingly testing promising technological platforms to improve caregiver-facing education and support interventions (Rickardsson, Stopforth, and Gillanders, 2020; Rietdijk, Togher, and Power, 2012; Spencer et al., 2019).

In this review, we identified studies that tested innovative and relatively novel approaches to TBI treatment and support, including technological interventions, such as virtual reality. Evidence development is in early stages, but extant research demonstrates promise that virtual reality may support motor and cognitive function (Cano Porras et al., 2018). In addition, computer-based cognitive retraining may support memory rehabilitation (Spreij et al., 2014). More broadly, digital approaches to care, including telehealth, may improve access and resources for people with mobility or functional limitations, people with comorbidities, the homebound, and those geographically distant from traditional care and rehabilitation centers (Zhou and Parmanto, 2019).

Limitations

The evidence map in Figure 5.2 was limited by the quality and clarity of evidence available in the systematic reviews. Individual studies included in the systematic reviews were of varying quality and high heterogeneity, so aggregate findings and conclusions were often vague, mixed, and uncertain. The nature of a review of systematic reviews (that is, an umbrella review) like the one we conducted may exclude individual relevant studies published after the included systematic reviews conducted their literature searches or that were excluded based on constrained systematic review inclusion criteria. This scenario is likely minimized because our umbrella review captured overlap of studies, evidence, and updates of the science as of July 2021. Furthermore, by using umbrella review methodology, we likely captured higher-quality science and interpretation in the primary studies that reached the threshold for inclusion in the systematic reviews that we subsequently included.

Conclusions

Evidence supports cognitive rehabilitation for cognitive outcomes, psychotherapy for psychological outcomes, behavioral interventions for social outcomes, occupational rehabilitation for occupational outcomes, and psychotherapy and behavioral interventions for PCS. Even so, most TBI research is conducted among the general adult population and often includes non-TBI neurological diagnoses that may result in imprecise or inaccurate efficacy of interventions to support veterans with TBI specifically. Innovations and traditional treatments for TBI show promise, but additional high-quality research in veteran populations is essential to understanding the most-effective interventions for improving outcomes after TBI.

Resources Available to Veterans with Traumatic Brain Injury

In this chapter, we present our analysis of the landscape of available resources, such as health care facilities and programs, that support TBI recovery for veterans or their caregivers. We identified and catalogued existing TBI resources from web and database searches and created a tool that allowed us to search these resources. Then, we mapped the location and availability of resources relative to where WWP alumni live, using five-digit zip code data.

Approach to Building a Database of Resources for Veterans with Traumatic Brain Injury

We used a two-pronged approach to identify institutions and programs for our database. We first implemented a Boolean search in Google based on keywords under three domains: TBI terms, treatment terms, and veteran-specific terms. We then searched broadly and with each U.S. state name to ensure that we identified programs across the United States. Figure 6.1 provides an overview of the search terms in each domain. The Boolean search queries combined all terms within domains using "or" statements and linked across domains 1 and 2 using "and" statements, and then again domains 1–3 using "and" statements to identify general

FIGURE 6.1
Search Terms

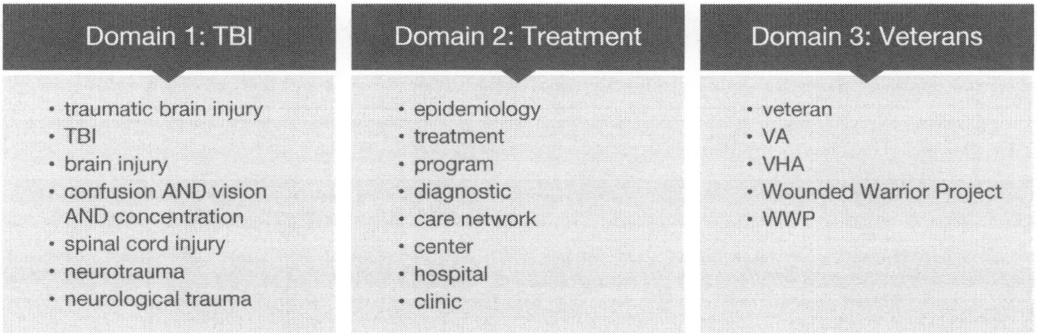

Domain 1: TBI	Domain 2: Treatment	Domain 3: Veterans
• traumatic brain injury • TBI • brain injury • confusion AND vision AND concentration • spinal cord injury • neurotrauma • neurological trauma	• epidemiology • treatment • program • diagnostic • care network • center • hospital • clinic	• veteran • VA • VHA • Wounded Warrior Project • WWP

programs and veteran-specific programs. Our goal was to identify more programs at this stage and then exclude ineligible programs on closer inspection, so our search terms were broad by design.

Second, we examined existing databases of TBI resources for veterans, including those from the Brain Injury Association of America (undated), Brainline (undated), and the National Institute of Child Health and Human Development (undated). We verified the information in those databases and abstracted other relevant information, such as program or organization address and phone number.

From these two approaches, we identified 1,450 entries from web searches and 17,824 from existing databases. We applied initial inclusion criteria to this list and retained only the entries that were one of the following types of resources:

- VA medical center or health system
- VA outpatient clinic that specifically listed TBI treatment or services on its website
- non-VA hospital that highlighted services for TBI on its website
- program or organization that provided TBI rehabilitation
- program or organization that provided TBI-specific counseling
- program or organization that provided services for family members of patients with brain injury.

After applying the initial inclusion criteria, we retained 6,729 entries for closer review and abstraction.

Development of the Geocoded Resource Database

To create our database showing where WWP alumni live in relation to TBI resources, we closely examined each entry to remove duplicates, obtained location information (address) for each entry, and abstracted relevant information about the types of services provided. We identified duplicates by sorting records on facility name to detect facilities with the same name and then visually inspecting other data items, including city and state, to identify facilities with similar names in different locations. Redundant records referring to the same resource were excluded.

Geocoding

The initial web-scraping and searching procedure yielded a variety of information that could be useful in locating facilities, including the facility name, street address, city, state, and zip code. A street address was initially collected for fewer than half of the records. We used a Python-coded script to send the available information for each record to Google's Geocoding API service, which was able to return a standardized address and geographic coordinates for more than 99 percent of the records. It was not possible to fully validate the returned locations, and for some facilities with only limited information available, the location might be incorrect. When we identified errors, we manually corrected those addresses. We excluded entries when the location was identified as being outside the United States.

Data Abstraction

In the next step, we manually reviewed the geocoded records for inclusion and data abstraction. We excluded resources that provided care only for children; were individuals (such as names of chaplains, therapists, or suicide prevention coordinators); were local offices of the National Association for Mental Illness or other programs that were broadly about trauma or neurology and did not reference TBI specifically; provided only legal aid services; or were duplicates of existing entries. We also excluded Vet Centers because they provide community-based counseling rather than TBI-specific treatment or resources.

Next, we abstracted information about the types of services provided by each resource. We categorized resources as follows:

- hospitals
- VA medical centers (including regional VA health systems)
- resources that offer veteran-specific services
- resources that offer physical health care
- resources that offer physical therapy
- resources that offer occupational therapy
- resources that offer speech therapy
- resources that offer mental health care
- resources that offer relationship support services
- resources that offer financial planning
- resources that offer employment programs
- resources that offer support groups
- resources that offer programs for caregivers and families.

During the abstraction process, we reconciled resource names further, identified additional duplicates, and identified many resources as not relevant. That process led to the exclusion of 4,371 resources. Nine additional resources were manually added. The final database included 2,325 TBI resources. We then built a tool programmed in RShiny that allowed us to search, map, filter, and link to the 2,325 resources identified. (For more information on RShiny, see Chang et al., 2021.)

Analysis of the Availability of Resources Relative to Where WWP Alumni Live

To determine how easily veterans who are engaged with WWP are able to access TBI resources, we mapped the driving time between WWP alumni's home zip codes and the zip codes of the resources included in our database. WWP provided RAND with data on all WWP alumni as of September 17, 2019 ($n = 133,469$ veterans). The data included information about demographics, military service history, health problems (including whether the veteran had sustained a TBI), and five-digit home zip code.

We geocoded the WWP data using ArcGIS Desktop version 10.6. Specifically, we geolocated the centroid of the five-digit home zip code for each veteran. We successfully geocoded zip codes for 98.2 percent (131,126 of 133,469) of the veterans in the WWP file. We calculated the minimum drive to each type of TBI resource (e.g., mental health care, caregiver program) from the centroid of the five-digit zip code. Using these data, we recorded the mean, median, and standard deviation (SD) for these minimum drive times. We also produced heat maps that graphically show the number of TBI resources that are within a 60-minute drive from the centroid of the zip code.

Findings

Among the 2,325 resources that we identified, 1,228 (54 percent) provided services for physical health, including physical therapy, occupational therapy, and speech therapy (but not all resources detailed the availability of these services) (Table 6.1). In addition, 1,257 (55 percent) provided services for mental health (many provided both physical and mental health services). Among physical and mental health providers, we identified 586 hospitals, including

TABLE 6.1
Number of Traumatic Brain Injury Resources, by Type

TBI Resource Category	Number of Resources
Hospital	586
VA medical center	174
Veteran-specific services	511
Physical health care	1,228
Physical therapy	476
Occupational therapy	460
Speech therapy	453
Mental health care	1,257
Relationship support services	487
Financial planning	246
Employment programs	391
Support groups	317
Programs for caregivers and families	741

NOTE: Additional resources may have offered these services but did not indicate it on their website.

174 VA medical centers, that provided specific treatment for TBI. About one-fourth of the resources (24 percent) provided primarily veteran-specific services. Some programs offered relationship support services (487), financial planning services (246), and employment programs (391). We identified 317 resources with support groups, and many resources (741) provided programs for caregivers and families.

Resources were distributed unevenly across the country, likely related to population density and veteran population density. For example, we identified 219 resources in Virginia and eight in the District of Columbia, yet we identified 19 resources in West Virginia, 21 in Arkansas, and 20 in Wyoming. States with the highest number of WWP alumni were some of the most populous in the country, including Texas, Florida, California, North Carolina, and Georgia (Figure 6.2).

Similarly, counties with the highest number of WWP alumni included Bexar, Texas (4,180); San Diego, California (3,194); El Paso, Colorado (2,842); Maricopa, Arizona (2,529); Cumberland, North Carolina (2,460); Harris, Texas (2,183); Duval, Florida (1,841); Bell, Texas (1,437); Montgomery, Tennessee (1,405); and Honolulu, Hawaii (1,367). Counties with the highest number of WWP alumni with TBI included Bexar, Texas (888); El Paso, Colorado (852); San Diego, California (702); Maricopa, Arizona (676); Cumberland, North Carolina (608); Harris, Texas (424); Montgomery, Tennessee (359); Bell, Texas (355); Los Angeles, California (350); and El Paso, Texas (343).

Table 6.2 reports the mean, median, and standard deviation for the minimum drive time in minutes from the centroid of a veteran's zip code to any TBI resource, as well as to the various types of TBI resources. The average minimum drive time to any TBI resource for WWP

FIGURE 6.2
States with the Largest Number of WWP Alumni

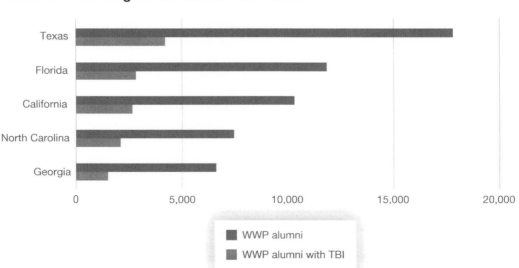

TABLE 6.2

Mean Drive Times to Traumatic Brain Injury Resources for WWP Alumni (in minutes)

TBI Resource Category	All WWP Alumni			WWP Alumni with TBI		
	Mean	Median	SD	Mean	Median	SD
Any TBI resource	35.47	26.11	29.92	31.73	22.31	28.08
Hospital	46.00	39.13	32.22	42.63	34.69	30.67
VA medical center	55.06	51.14	33.05	52.42	47.50	31.95
Veteran-specific services	47.99	40.68	33.48	44.52	36.20	31.93
Physical health care	40.04	31.39	31.17	36.54	26.91	29.60
Occupational therapy	48.55	41.50	33.61	45.40	37.59	32.07
Physical therapy	48.14	40.98	33.38	45.12	37.37	31.84
Speech therapy	48.09	40.89	33.45	45.0	37.05	31.90
Mental health care	39.68	30.74	31.13	35.99	26.46	29.42
Relationship support services	47.07	39.14	32.92	44.06	35.51	31.51
Employment programs	49.29	42.24	33.91	45.96	38.03	32.44
Financial planning	51.01	44.14	33.81	48.25	40.65	32.47
Support groups	50.16	43.88	33.33	47.48	40.54	31.87
Program for caregivers and families	46.34	38.18	33.39	42.74	33.80	31.82

NOTE: In this analysis, for the all WWP alumni category, we used zip codes that contained at least one WWP veteran. For the WWP alumni with TBI category, we used zip codes that contained at least one WWP veteran who self-reported having TBI.

alumni from the centroid of their zip code was 35.47 minutes (median = 26.11, SD = 29.92). The average hospital and VA medical center was 46.00 (median = 39.13, SD = 32.22) and 55.06 (median = 51.14, SD = 33.05) minutes away, respectively. Veteran-specific services were located within a mean drive time of 48.00 minutes (median = 40.68, SD = 33.48). More-tailored programs for occupational therapy, physical therapy, speech therapy, relationship support services, employment programs, financial planning, and support groups, as well as programs for caregivers and families, were located similar distances from the centroid of the veteran's zip code.

Of all the five-digit zip codes in the United States, 56.71 percent had WWP alumni ($n = 17,273$), and 35.01 percent had WWP alumni who reported having TBI when enrolling in WWP. We calculated the mean number of TBI resources within a 30- and 60-minute drive of WWP alumni and of WWP alumni with TBI (using the centroid of their reported home zip codes).

We also calculated the mean number of VA medical centers within a 30- and 60-minute drive of these groups. We found that, on average, there were 0.24 (SD = 0.50) VA medical centers within a 30-minute drive and 0.62 (SD = 0.88) VA medical centers within a 60-minute drive of WWP alumni. Figure 6.3 is a heat map depicting the number of VA medical centers within a 60-minute drive of WWP alumni's zip codes throughout the United States. Compared with all WWP alumni, those with TBI had slightly more geographic access to a VA medical center: On average, there were 0.26 (SD = 0.51) VA medical centers within a 30-minute drive and 0.66 (SD = 0.87) VA medical centers within a 60-minute drive of veterans with TBI. Our results also indicate that WWP alumni had relatively less access to VA medical centers than to non-VA hospitals that provided TBI-specific treatment, but veterans with TBI had somewhat better access to these services than veterans without TBI did.

Next, we assessed whether WWP alumni had geographic access to TBI resources that provided veteran-specific services. We found that, on average, WWP alumni had 0.91 (SD = 2.06) veteran-specific TBI resources within a 30-minute drive and 2.35 (SD = 3.90) within a 60-minute drive. Figure 6.4 shows the variation in geographic access to veteran-specific TBI resources. The average number of veteran-specific TBI resources close to WWP

FIGURE 6.3
VA Medical Centers Within a 60-Minute Drive of WWP Alumni

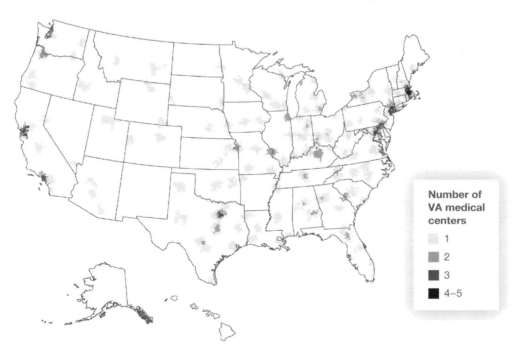

NOTE: White spaces are all census tracts where there is no VA medical center within a 60-minute drive.

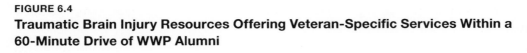

FIGURE 6.4

Traumatic Brain Injury Resources Offering Veteran-Specific Services Within a 60-Minute Drive of WWP Alumni

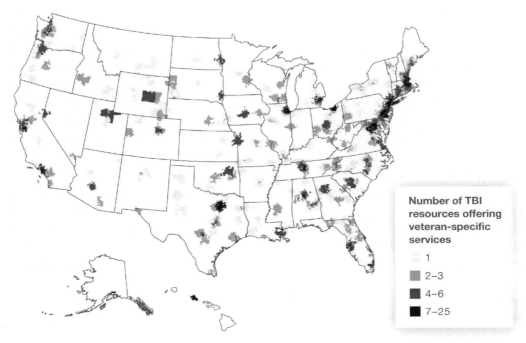

NOTE: White spaces are all census tracts where there are no TBI resources offering veteran-specific services within a 60-minute drive.

alumni with TBI were similar: 0.99 (SD = 2.07) within a 30-minute drive and 2.55 (SD = 3.84) within a 60-minute drive. The results indicate that most WWP alumni appeared to have multiple options for TBI resources with veteran-specific services within a 60-minute drive of the centroid of their home zip code.

For additional analyses, see Appendix D.

Summary

Through a systematic search and screening process, we identified and categorized 2,325 TBI resources across the United States. These resources include medical facilities and other organizations that serve veterans by providing physical health care, mental health care, and targeted services needed for TBI rehabilitation.

We found that the average drive time to a TBI resource was about 30 minutes for WWP alumni, although this depended on the type of resource. For example, accessing a VA medical center required a longer drive time (up to 60 minutes). WWP alumni had faster geographic access to physical health care services than to mental health care services.

Although the analyses presented in this chapter offer insights into geographic access for WWP alumni with TBI, there are some limitations. First, our database of resources is not completely comprehensive of all locations where a veteran could receive treatment for TBI. For example, there are 6,000 hospitals in the United States, and most have some TBI services. Our database includes only 586 hospitals, including all VA medical centers and other hospitals that came up in a search for TBI. We did not include the numerous VA clinics that may offer support for TBI or redirect individuals to other TBI care. Although we tried to be systematic, there are certainly resources that we may have missed and others that may have been included that no longer offer relevant services, given our web-based search process and the risk of websites not being updated. At the same time, many resources have limited information online about the services that they provide, so it is possible that the resources in our database may provide more services than what we found.

Second, we calculated each of the minimum drive time distances using the centroid of the WWP veteran's zip code. Future work should perform similar analyses using the household address of a WWP veteran, if possible. This would be a more accurate representation of geographic access because some zip codes cover a large geographic area. Third, although we calculated geographic access to resources, we did not assess the capacity of those resources. A resource might offer many of these services for WWP alumni with TBI, but it might not have available slots to do so. Fourth, our data on WWP alumni with TBI are from self-reports. Such data may be subject to bias. Finally, although we calculated the minimum distance to a TBI resource, we did not capture other measures that would affect access, such as what forms of insurance are accepted as payment.

Despite these limitations, we successfully identified a variety of resources across the country that serve veterans with a focus on TBI needs. We were also able to create maps that show where services are clustered and where they are lacking, which allows us to identify potential gaps in access.

Perspectives on Addressing the Long-Term Impacts of Traumatic Brain Injury Among Veterans

In this chapter, we detail findings from interviews with subject-matter experts, including researchers and clinicians from a variety of settings (e.g., VA, academic medical centers, non-VA community-based care settings) and scientific advisers. This qualitative research complements the evidence, and knowledge gaps, highlighted in Chapters Two and Five by contextualizing some of the on-the-ground challenges and opportunities surrounding the diagnosis of, treatment of, and continued care for TBI among post-9/11 veterans.

Approach to Interviews with Subject-Matter Experts

Sampling

We created a convenience sample of U.S.-based public and private experts and stakeholders by identifying key authors in the literature review, recognized clinical experts who serve on national consensus committees, directors of brain trauma centers both within VA and in private treatment centers, and leaders of TBI consortia. In addition, we consulted with WWP staff regarding experts whose perspectives they sought. We also used a respondent-driven sampling approach (i.e., "snowball" sampling) to contact additional experts.

We identified and reached out to 21 experts and sent a one-time follow-up via email. Potential interviewees were provided with a brief description of the study aims and an explanation of consent. The final sample included 16 interviewees across the United States with the following areas of expertise: neuroscience, psychiatry, neuropsychology, physiology, psychology, neurology, pathology, internal medicine, vascular surgery, nuclear medicine, rehabilitation medicine, recreation therapy, and epidemiology. In addition, several experts were serving or had served in the U.S. military.

Interview Protocol

We designed a comprehensive, semi-structured interview protocol to elicit expert perspectives on typical issues faced by veterans with differing degrees of TBI (mild, moderate, or severe), common comorbidities associated with TBI, the state of the evidence linking TBI to chronic conditions (e.g., diabetes, early-onset dementia, cardiovascular issues), the impact of patient characteristics on care delivery, the role of trauma-informed care, barriers and facilitators to providing care, the evidence base on clinical approaches to treating TBI, the evidence base linking TBI to long-term disorders, and overall perspectives on how to improve the state of the science and treatment with respect to TBI in the U.S. military and veteran population. The protocol was co-created by members of our research team with expertise in the field. The semi-structured interview protocol allowed for respondents to elaborate on key areas pertinent to their areas of expertise.

Data Analysis

The data analysis for these interviews followed the same procedures outlined in Chapter Four.

Findings

Military-related TBI, along with its related sequalae of complications, is a relatively recent phenomenon. Although service members certainly experienced TBIs before 9/11, shifts in the style of tactical warfare, including an increase in exposure to explosive blasts, and advances in protective equipment, which have saved lives, have arguably contributed to a greater prevalence of TBI. As an invisible wound of war, the public health ramifications of TBI were not readily recognized at the start of the 21st-century Iraq and Afghanistan conflicts. However, growing attention to the issue as it relates to force readiness, coupled with increasing public awareness of sport-related concussions, has placed TBI research and care delivery in a state of growth and development.

Experts contributed insights from a multitude of vantage points, such as military-, VA-, and community-based (i.e., private) care; basic science and translational research; clinical research; epidemiological research; and implementation science. Perspectives varied on key debates, such as the risk for accelerated aging among those with TBI, and disagreement in describing the work of others was at times rather spirited. Despite these differences, experts outlined several areas to advance the state of research and care to address the long-term consequences of TBI.

The findings we report in this chapter are organized by interrelated themes. The presentation of the findings is intended to reflect the variety of responses expressed by experts in the field and not to emphasize any particular viewpoint.

Diagnosing Traumatic Brain Injury

The lack of clarity surrounding TBI trajectories begins with veterans' difficulty in recalling the event that caused the injury—or, in many cases, the series of injuries that took place—and the severity of the injury or injuries.

Clinicians described the fundamental issues surrounding how a diagnosis of a TBI is made and how to differentiate among mild, moderate, and severe cases. Loss of consciousness is generally used as a benchmark between mild and moderate to severe cases. Brain scans may not be indicative of the severity of an injury. As a clinician of veteran populations noted, brain scans in the acute post-injury phase are rarely indicative of one's prognosis, even when brain bleeds or hemorrhaging is present. Another clinician added that a person's subjective reporting of symptoms after acute injury does not always match neurological differences in brain scans.

The vagueness surrounding a diagnosis (i.e., whether a TBI was sustained) was most often applied to mild cases, and, even then, questions remained about the cumulative impact of multiple mild TBIs. As a clinician working with veteran populations explained,

> How to define repetitive concussions is a moving target. I believe that, based on the data, a single concussion has a good prognosis. We don't know about concentration over a particular time period. Military personnel, when deployed, could very easily sustain multiple TBIs over a short period of time. Is there a key number of TBIs where we start to see a difference? Is it three or five TBIs? Or is it anything greater than one? Doing assessments very much after the fact and getting retrospective data is a challenge both clinically and for research purposes.

Another clinician added, "There is some work among those who have had three or more concussions that shows greater subjective distress, headaches, emotional difficulties, and PTSD symptoms but no objective neurocognitive and neuropsychological differences." Clinicians were split on how definitive the delineations between mild and moderate or severe TBI are; one clinician asserted that, although a more severe case will almost undoubtedly result in the need for acute treatment, "you almost have to be a specialist on TBI to get it reasonably right, and this can even be difficult for clinicians with decades of experience." Another clinician with military experience explained,

> If we're in combat and we're near a blast, and it is enough to cause some type of other bodily injury or cause someone to stop breathing, those are things that are going to be treated right away to save that person's life. But we forget that there was enough energy in the blast to eviscerate somebody. But because they come into care unconscious, we automatically assumed that it was the shock or hypomania and not a brain injury. So, a traumatic brain injury, you could have a concussion and, by definition, your CT [computed tomography] scan is normal, so you may not get a diagnosis of concussion.

Veterans may also have poor recall of events, with a bias toward recalling extreme blast events in combat. As a veteran-turned-researcher explained, "If you asked guys if they were exposed to a blast, they're only going to think about an IED. I wouldn't think about any other potential blasts. This makes it really tricky for anyone looking for causation; veterans don't have an objective record."

Clinicians described using symptom duration to retroactively evaluate the severity of a TBI; some asserted that, if symptoms subside within 30 days, a soldier has suffered a concussion, but if symptoms persist for 60 to 90 days, the condition is likely PCS. Another clinician parsed out acute versus chronic conditions by stating that, if someone does not recover cognitively, behaviorally, and functionally to where they were pre-injury within 12 months, it should be considered a chronic condition.

Then there is the issue of delays in recognizing a TBI that are unique to the military. Because a TBI is an invisible wound, a service member can suffer several such injuries before a TBI diagnosis is made or treatment is given—a theme that was commonly endorsed by veterans in our sample (see Chapter Four). Despite having symptoms of a TBI, soldiers may be unwilling to retreat from a combat zone in an effort to fulfill the mission at hand. Furthermore, as noted by experts who had served or were actively serving in the military, commanders may also overlook potential cases of TBI in favor of completing a mission. As one clinician described,

> If I can still do this and I can point my weapon system in the right direction, I could have a lost arm, but we're still going to complete the mission. . . . If I get a laceration, I can put a tourniquet on, and maybe I am good for another hour until medical care arrives. We're still trying to figure out the situation *right now*. If I get bonked on the head and I have a concussion, but they can't evacuate immediately, what can you do?

Experts mentioned that, prior to 2007, there was a reluctance in the military to readily screen for TBI and other invisible wounds (e.g., PTSD) out of concern that it would affect force readiness. An influx of veterans with TBI and co-occurring PTSD prompted a protocol to screen service members for TBI. But, as another clinician described from the front lines, enacting real-time screening was not always practical or acceptable:

> It was the line leader's responsibility to report those people who were in motor vehicle accidents, bopped their heads, if they were within 100 meters of a blast. With this aspect of team leadership, a leader, whether it's a sergeant or a lieutenant, should be the person who knows their people the best. So, if someone wasn't acting right, that would also prompt an evaluation. We got a lot of pushback though because everyone assumed that screening equaled diagnosis. So, once we educated that it was a screening process, we got better numbers.

The inconsistency in screening for and diagnosing TBIs is further compounded by the fact that symptoms of TBI can mirror other conditions. One clinician explained that TBI can often be mistaken for musculoskeletal cervical segmental dysfunction and injuries to the cervical spine that can (like TBI) result in persistent headaches. Far more common, however, is the co-occurrence of PTSD and other mental health issues, including depression and anxiety.

Traumatic Brain Injury and Comorbid Conditions

Mental and Behavioral Health Issues

Veterans of Operation Enduring Freedom and Operation Iraqi Freedom who experienced TBI often present with co-occurring PTSD, which is often related to adverse experiences in the military or in combat. Both conditions are considered invisible wounds of war, and both can create a suite of challenges in a soldier's life, but the military has deemed only TBI as a potential qualifying injury for a Purple Heart. A clinician with experience on the front lines remarked, "It's a strange conundrum that PTSD—and depression and anxiety—are not medical problems, but TBI is, and then of course you have that overlap across them all." In fact, experts noted that symptoms of PTSD are often mistaken for TBI but that there is a bias toward ascribing symptoms to TBI as opposed to PTSD, perhaps given the stigmatization of the latter. A clinician described preliminary research showing that veterans who ascribed at least some of their prolonged symptoms to PTSD and not exclusively to their TBI were more likely to engage in treatment than those who attributed their symptoms to TBI.

Providers are not always equipped to treat co-occurring PTSD and TBI; some even considered patients with TBI to be unable to engage in some PTSD treatments. "Clinically, these are challenging patients," as one clinician noted. "Multimodal treatments can be important and effective. Just because someone has a history of TBI does not mean that they cannot benefit from" prolonged exposure therapy or cognitive processing therapy.

Another clinician spoke of "clear evidence supporting the link among brain changes that can contribute to risk for depression within five years of a TBI." The same clinician mentioned the links between migraines and depression risk, poor sleep hygiene and depression risk, and diabetes and depression risk.

Metabolic and Cardiovascular Disorders

Clinicians and researchers mentioned the links between TBI and weight gain through neuroendocrine alterations, although the exact pathways are still being identified. These neuroendocrine functions can increase risk for diabetes and cardiovascular issues. As a clinician noted,

> What influences the rate of cognitive and physical deterioration is yet to be known. One other complicating factor in this equation is the amount of weight gain that occurs in these individuals. This clearly impacts the physical ability and influences cardiovascular problems, which can further influence deterioration in mental ability for those who had a TBI. We don't know how this may be interrelated, but we can assume that we are going to see increasing medical support needs for these individuals because of the constellation of injuries and medical problems that accrue as they age.

He continued, "Given that we are two decades down the pike from the start of the [post-9/11] wars, these are issues that we are going to start seeing now, and that is why this needs to be studied *now*."

Chronic Traumatic Encephalopathy, Dementia, and Alzheimer's Disease

When subject-matter experts were prompted to discuss long-term issues among veterans who sustained TBIs, the overwhelming topic of discussion was the potential but contentious link between TBI and the risk for CTE, early-onset dementia, and Alzheimer's disease. Experts were polarized on this topic; in fact, one clinician warned,

> Without being overdramatic, I'm suggesting that we may be facing a tsunami [of early-onset cognitive decline]. I don't want to be overdramatic about it, but we've learned certain things from some of the preliminary neural pathway studies. We know that we've got a cohort of warriors that have suffered TBI or repetitive TBI in the special operations community, and this is why I think we need to jump on this to better understand what the evolving story is.

This standpoint was countered by another clinical expert on concussions, who noted,

> Things are not nearly as bad as the advocates think they are when it comes to TBI and aging, in my view. Advocates that want to talk about the sky is falling and you really need to deal with this enormous problem that's going to be a tsunami of a problem in the future. My concern is about dementia in general as our population ages. That concern for me is considerably far, far greater than my concern for veterans who have had a mild traumatic brain injury at some point in their life. It's very easy to get caught up in the hype of, "oh my gosh, I played high school football" or "I served in the United States military and I'm going to develop a deadly brain disease at some point in the future." I would say, "Where's the scientific evidence for that?"

Several other clinicians and researchers tempered the possible "tsunami" or the lack thereof by cautioning that there are insufficient data and considerable limitations in study designs to assess the association between TBI and the suite of neurological and cognitive issues. One epidemiologist who has long been tracking the association between mild TBI and dementia added, "We have a long way to go. There's too much junk published in medical journals, and they don't pay attention to study design—case reports are seen as causation. If a clinician is not educated in research, those case reports look like the canary in the coal mine."

Other clinicians of primarily veteran populations underscored the fact that many risk factors for dementia and Alzheimer's disease are modifiable, such as obesity and smoking. Another clinician-researcher added,

> The question, in my mind, is how much of this is the immediate impacts of a TBI versus what gets termed "early-onset dementia"? We have to be very careful with these terminologies. It doesn't necessarily mean this is an early neurodegenerative disease. All it could mean is somebody has a significant cognitive decline. But guess what? They could rebound from that.

As noted earlier, how to delineate the acute, recoverable cases from the chronic cases is unknown. And, although the data point to some links between TBI and accelerated aging of the brain, one expert who elaborated on underlying misunderstandings of risk added, "I'm not talking about accelerated aging at 45; instead of getting these things when you're 75, maybe you're going to be 73. We're not talking decades." These overestimations of risk are further compounded by the fact that one's underlying risk is difficult to quantify, given the underlying complications of diagnosing TBI. This was echoed by a CTE researcher, who explained that issues with measurement and a patient's recall of the severity of the TBI, in addition to the lack of clarity on how such comorbidities as PTSD factor into risk, make establishing correlations between TBI and CTE murky. One CTE researcher also noted that a PTSD brain bank is showing a clear overlap among PTSD and CTE, but there are "probably some other confounders in there as well. Clinically, it's very difficult to disentangle—that is, until we have a biomarker of TBI," a feat that is well into development, at least for more-severe TBIs. This researcher added, "We certainly see substance use disorder as a way to cope with TBI and PTSD, which can lead to a lack of focus, impulsivity, depression, and sleep issues— all things where the brain doesn't seem to be in control anymore. Does it make CTE worse? We don't know." Another clinician reiterated this point, stating, "The key is not only dissecting out the specifics of what might be accelerated dementia as a result of TBI, but it really will be important to tell a story about these associated morbidities that result in greater clinical and physical needs and loss of quality of life as wounded warriors age."

CTE is a diagnosis of exclusion and can be diagnosed only post-mortem. Nevertheless, additional CTE researchers focusing on data from brain banks assert the presence of a clear dose-response, at least among football players in the United States (adding that data are lacking for military and veteran populations). Assisting this process is the fact that the supposed "massive denial" (as one interviewee put it) of the link between TBI and CTE is lifting. As one expert noted, "Pretty much everyone now understands that it is an issue, but it's not in the military's best interest to focus on this since it would put a damper on people joining the military." Still, leading researchers on CTE were quick to note that "most veterans will *not* have CTE," and "CTE does not happen from a single TBI, or even well-spaced mild TBIs." But, as for the link between repetitive head traumas, "the evidence is there. It's real; it's in peer-reviewed, high-level journals." Without more data in brain banks (i.e., more donations to brain banks from veterans), a biomarker for TBI, and increased insights into controlling for confounding conditions, the link between TBI and CTE may remain unclear.

Given these complexities, conveying the trajectories of TBI treatment and the management of comorbidities to military and veteran populations and their caregivers presents its own challenges. In the next section, we present clinician perspectives on the delivery of care to military and veteran populations.

Treatment for Traumatic Brain Injury Among Veterans

Clinicians who treat veterans spoke about veterans' general concerns with cognitive and physical decline in the years following a TBI. These clinicians underscored the importance of defining and understanding care needs among those with polytrauma, such as TBI and PTSD. Care delivery for TBI is often concentrated in specific programming. For example, the current VA Polytrauma/TBI System of Care generally consists of visits every four to six weeks, then every two to three months, for a total of six to eight visits. But, given patients' risk for long-term chronic health issues, clinicians emphasized the importance of engaging veterans (and their caregivers) in long-term wellness through integrated models of care. Families and caregivers can be a critical aspect of promoting long-term health and setting realistic, optimistic expectations. A clinician specializing in care for veterans added,

> The family needs to understand what recovery is about and that the patient doesn't hate them and isn't a "different human being." They're someone who has a disorder just like alcoholism, obesity, all these kinds of things. It's not a death sentence! It's a condition that with the right family support, professional support, vocational supports, a patient is going to have a very good chance of wonderful recovery. Or, worst-case scenario, they're not going to be exactly the same as before, but they're going to have a very productive life.

In describing knowledge gaps, another clinician tempered this more optimistic view for moderate and severe TBI cases:

> Neuroscience continues to be the Wild West of medicine. We're learning things every day about the regenerative powers of the brain, but also about the crossover between structural problems in the brain, mental health issues, particularly when the frontal lobe has been injured and there's a loss of executive function. The point I'm making is that there's a lot to be discovered about how often we treat these individuals and what the eventual outcome will be. As people with moderate and severe TBI age, there is potential for cognitive decline. The issue is, how accelerated will it be? And then what are the other comorbidities that might even accelerate it further? The issue is often you can't tell them specifically what their outcome is going to be in five or ten years because I don't think we know it.

Building the evidence base will be important for enhancing existing understandings of the links among TBI, comorbidities, and long-term cognitive outcomes. The need for prolonged care and monitoring prompted one clinician to suppose that TBI should, in some cases, be considered a chronic condition:

> Some people will recover, but some may not quite fully recover. The emphasis is primarily on the acute TBI and then people kind of don't pay much attention after that. TBI is not always but *sometimes* a chronic condition. If we can start to see it that way, then I think the connections with aging can make a lot of sense. It's very hard to communicate risks to people, so somehow communicating that this is not a doom at all to veterans is important.

To the clinicians we interviewed, communicating the fact that most TBIs are mild cases, that symptoms generally resolve within a year post-injury, and that early-onset dementia is in no way a foregone conclusion is as important as urging veterans to continue to engage in physical health, mental health, and wellness long after their injury. One clinician noted,

> You need to stay in touch with your doctor, you need to have regular visits, and you also want to really try to take care of yourself, work on your sleep hygiene, get more physical activity, take care of your depression, lose some weight, and all of these things. And I think that just like we do those things to try and prevent dementia, these are things that you would want to start teaching people about early, so they maximize their aging.

This was echoed by another clinician specializing in veterans' care, who stated, "The real key is active engagement and active participation in a treatment plan. TBI care is not going to be chronologically driven. How do you promote active engagement? It's trying to figure out what's health care and what is wellness." Promoting wellness, as another clinician reiterated, would help veterans "pivot away from what we currently think is a tsunami of cognitive impairment." In short, clinicians highlighted the importance of addressing quality of life and mental health, tracking cardiovascular and metabolic health, encouraging patients to avoid alcohol and substances, and clearly conveying that health-promoting behaviors and time can help resolve adverse symptoms post-TBI.

Clinicians also mentioned the differences between civilian and veteran populations' experiences with TBI. One clinician focused on the fact that "the high incidence of co-occurring PTSD and TBI is vastly different than in the civilian population. Having providers that are aware of the potential exposures and challenges with deployment is critical." This segued into the particular advantages of seeking care from VA; one clinician working in the system described those advantages as the "providers' ability to work effectively," adding, "The time to provide interdisciplinary care isn't reimbursed at a high enough rate to incentivize in the private sector." VA also provides training to community-based (i.e., non-VA) providers to build military cultural competency, but, according to those familiar with the program, it has been underutilized. In addition, although we interviewed community-based providers who provide military- and veteran-specific services, such programming is not widely available and often requires veterans to travel to receive care.

Whether this type of interdisciplinary treatment for TBI and related comorbidities is accessible at VA sites that do not offer specific polytrauma programming is unclear. However, clinicians who serve military populations cautioned that, as the Operation Enduring Freedom and Operation Iraqi Freedom conflicts come to an end, interdisciplinary services that combine vestibular, neurological, psychological, physical therapy, and occupational therapy support are being "farmed out to primary care," and "mental and behavioral health services are severely unmanned," with "VA providers working themselves to death against a huge demand." Thus, there is a need to enhance interdisciplinary care and the resources necessary to make comprehensive, long-term care possible throughout the VA system.

Future Research Directions and Innovation

Subject-matter experts were asked about how they would move the needle on long-term outcomes for TBI. Unsurprisingly, experts put forth several suggestions that coalesced around research initiatives, augmented resources, and reconfigurations of existing systems of care. Experts all agreed that much work needs to be done, some praised the gains in basic science and clinical delivery, and others expressed some frustration with "not having a lot to show for" the boost in investments made in TBI since 2007.

Increasing Research Collaboration and Data Integration

To begin, researchers noted that funding for research collaboration and data integration is constrained, and there is competition for these funds, which has had the unintended consequence of creating silos of research groups that are not always primed for cross-dialogue and shared findings. There are, however, several collaborative research networks, such as the Traumatic Brain Injury Center of Excellence (through DoD's Military Health System), the Transforming Research and Clinical Knowledge in Traumatic Brain Injury (TRACK-TBI) study, and the Collaborative European NeuroTrauma Effectiveness Research in TBI (CENTER-TBI) study. Researchers questioned the degree to which the individual study consortia are in communication. Given the multifaceted impacts of TBI and the variety of disciplines needed to fully evaluate the issue, more collaboration across centers could be beneficial. One clinician and researcher said that doing so could help standardize definitions of pathology in the brain and parse out the impacts of TBI versus common co-occurring conditions, such as PTSD. Another clinician of veteran populations added that more collaboration across the DoD Traumatic Brain Injury Center of Excellence and the VA National Center for PTSD could bring about better insights into providing care for veterans with both conditions. In addition, such collaboration could streamline the quality of care that is delivered across VA sites.

Experts overwhelmingly discussed that the study of long-term issues from TBI is fraught with limitations in the underlying data. This is a common issue when seeking to understand a complex health condition, as with TBI among veterans, but it has become particularly weighty in light of concerns that TBI might cause early cognitive decline. Experts from all vantage points were quick to point out uncertainties in their areas of expertise on account of incomplete data, but they also mentioned opportunities for improvement. In addition, there are ongoing epidemiological research efforts in this space; for example, the Trajectories of Resilience, Community, and Health Lab at the University of Utah is building a data repository on long-term outcomes following military experiences. Building these data sets—and enacting evidence-based actions on account of those findings—will be an important goal going forward.

Challenges of diagnosis aside, syncing various systems in which the incidence of a TBI is captured—including systems from VA, the Military Health System, and community-based care—would be foundational for gaining a more accurate assessment of the magnitude of TBI among post-9/11 veterans. As was discussed in Chapter Four, veterans described having sometimes endured several TBIs before a more severe event with multiple injuries occurred. Hence, there may be issues in under- and overreporting of TBIs. As one military clinician noted, "Because the systems are not linked, the same TBI event can get captured multiple times and appear as though it was several events." Another clinician with extensive experience in both DoD and VA strongly supported cross-department capabilities and one-stop personnel screening processes that can rectify gaps within the information transfer between DoD and VA. Yet another clinician with extensive military experience spoke of the added layer of complexity of collating data from veterans who seek community-based care. At present, there is no requirement to submit medical records that were created outside of DoD and VA systems. Strengthening the quality and interoperability of the data sets of TBI-related acute and long-term impacts would be an imperative for understanding the related issues and the opportunities to provide better care among this population.

In a broader sense, there is a need to increase the quality of published data representing the general population as well. Existing data sets have been limited by not controlling for confounding variables; that is, the evidence base does not always account for such factors as one's alcohol and substance use, PTSD, or sleep hygiene in evaluating the association between TBI and such outcomes as dementia. Making a more concerted effort to follow veterans with TBI throughout their lives, and in turn capturing long-term functional and behavioral data, would allow significant strides in better understanding the ever-elusive association between TBI and long-term cognitive outcomes and could drive developments in precision medicine of treatment and prognoses.

Building More-Robust Data Sets

The diversity among post-9/11 veterans is not well represented in existing data sets. For example, research scientists and clinicians pointed out that very little is known about differences across sex, gender, race, and ethnicity. Given that post-9/11 veterans are the most diverse cohort of veterans in history (National Center for Veterans Analysis and Statistics, 2018), the field could use subanalyses across different demographic groups to better understand the trajectories and care needs of all veterans. Clinicians well versed in the military also noted that, because special operations forces have endured intense training and combat exposure (much of which is classified), this drives the need to understand their particular cognitive trajectories following TBI.

Enhancing brain banks among veterans would be one way to better understand the link between TBI and CTE. For one neuroscientist, "The best near-term investment we can make in the next decade would be getting more brain donations from veterans." The clinician added that, of 200 veterans in the brain bank, only one-third experienced their primary TBI exposure through military service. Other experts promoting the implementation of technology to measure blast gauge data added that brain banks could be synced with long-term blast exposure data to facilitate a better understanding of the dose-response relationship in brain health and TBI. An epidemiologist noted, however, that brain banks may not paint a complete picture, because consent to an autopsy may create a biased sample. Other clinicians cautioned that an overemphasis on devoting resources to brain banks may detract from the fact that there are real opportunities to intervene and improve the mental and physical health of veterans with TBI now, and those opportunities could get overlooked if the focus is on gleaning information post-mortem. However, one could argue that these goals need not be mutually exclusive.

Implementing Emerging Technologies

Several experts highlighted an opportunity to have health systems leverage emerging digital technologies "now that the home can serve as the first and last line of care." For instance, veterans could employ (1) wearable devices that can track aerobic exercise or sleep or (2) home-based digital support technologies that can track and respond to declines in cognitive function. Additionally, the rapid pivot to implement telehealth during the COVID-19 pandemic proved that great feats can be possible, but "now the system has to be retrofitted to really support it," as one clinician noted. Some of these shifts are already in progress; for example, VA is in the process of implementing assistance technology devices that are linked to cloud-based infrastructure. According to a VA clinician, "This has forced VA to be more modern and work through issues so that veterans have access to the latest technology." These system reconfigurations to implement novel technologies, synchronize data systems, and institute long-term care and wellness programming for veterans will require sustained funding from a coalition of efforts; in other words, funding likely should not be shouldered exclusively by VA, and discretionary funding from Congress may not be sufficient.

Providing Holistic Healing for Veterans

Experts described the need to move beyond the approach that is often ascribed to government agencies, which, according to one clinician, is to "administer benefits according to certain scales and statutes." These experts suggested moving toward approaches that WWP and similar organizations strive to take, which, in the words of one clinician, is to

> make these wounded warriors whole, not only physiologically, physically, and functionally, but also to evaluate how they integrate with their family unit and reintegrate into employment opportunities. . . . What needs to be done is really a specific kind of clinical assessment to assist with a better understanding of how these individuals will age and what support is still needed in society.

Summary

Subject-matter experts offered valuable insights into the complex fields of treating and researching TBI. Experts reiterated the complexities of providing a timely diagnosis of TBI and pinning down its severity. In addition, they described that those who sustained a TBI in the early years of the Operation Enduring Freedom and Operation Iraqi Freedom conflicts may not have been diagnosed, given that regular screening was mandated only after 2007.

Clinicians and researchers noted that experiencing TBI presents an increased risk, albeit modest, for several disorders. Although there were disagreements over the magnitude of this risk, all experts agreed that confounding comorbid conditions (e.g., PTSD) and ambiguity over the number and severity of TBIs make it nearly impossible to make definitive statements about risk for downstream health issues or the best ways to address or mitigate risk for these health issues. This ambiguity was mirrored in our two literature reviews on long-term health issues associated with TBI and interventions to address them, described in Chapters Two and Five, respectively. All of the interviewed experts reinforced the importance of promoting wellness and active engagement in care not only for TBI but also for common comorbid conditions, such as PTSD.

Furthermore, experts described several areas that could advance the state of the science and the delivery of care for veterans who sustained a TBI. Across the board, they underscored the need to solve the limitations in the underlying data on veterans with TBI. Those limitations could be mitigated by better syncing of data systems across DoD and the VHA, as well as by tracking veterans more concertedly and longitudinally. The experts also described a need for more collaboration across different research camps within TBI and for closer research efforts to understand the links between TBI and PTSD. Enhancing brain banks would also likely advance understanding of key issues surrounding TBI and brain health. Where possible, employing telehealth technologies, which was swiftly started during the COVID-19 pandemic, could further close gaps in accessing care.

CHAPTER EIGHT

Conclusions and Recommendations

The wars in Iraq and Afghanistan redefined the nature of combat, the demographics of those in combat, the frequency of deployments, the visible and invisible wounds sustained, and the care and services delivered to service members and veterans long after returning from war and separating from the military. Two decades after the wars began, the United States is facing the challenge of how to provide care to the veterans who sustained injuries during their voluntary enlistments and service.

One central health-related consequence of the post-9/11 wars is the high proportion of service members and veterans who sustained a TBI. TBI can be a particularly complex condition in military and veteran populations because of the difficulty of its diagnosis; the variety of physical, metabolic, cognitive, and behavioral detriments that it can create or exacerbate; and its interconnectedness with other disorders, such as PTSD. In this report, we explored known long-term outcomes related to TBI, as well as present-day challenges that veterans and their families face in navigating their daily lives and in accessing care. In sum, we focused on how to improve care and services over the long term for veterans experiencing ongoing disability and problems subsequent to TBI.

Summary of Findings

After the introduction to this report, we reviewed the state of the evidence of long-term (i.e., post-acute) issues associated with TBI (Chapter Two). Long-term outcomes, including psychological conditions (e.g., depression and suicidality), were generally worse for those who had experienced one or more TBIs than for those who had not. There is also evidence that TBI can increase the risk of certain neurodegenerative health conditions, such as ALS, Alzheimer's disease, and Parkinson's disease. There is evidence that initially poor cognitive outcomes in such areas as attention improve over time and can continue to improve for several years after TBI. However, much of the research is complicated by a relatively low-quality evidence base and is limited by selection and recall biases. Furthermore, the evidence on long-term outcomes specific to military and veteran populations with TBI is scant. This was particularly the case for evidence on the long-term cognitive impacts of TBI, which were a critical challenge for many veterans and caregivers whom we interviewed (Chapter Four).

We then turned to data collected from WWP's Annual Alumni Survey to explore associations between WWP alumni who self-reported sustaining a head injury during their military service and various outcomes, compared with associations for WWP alumni without a head injury (Chapter Three). These data showed that those with a head injury differed in important ways from those without a head injury. Head injury was more prevalent among men, the medically retired, and veterans from the Army and Marine Corps. Those with a head injury were also more severely impaired, had higher disability ratings and more comorbidities, and relied more on caregivers. They were less likely to be employed, although they had similar rates of enrollment in school. Multivariable analyses that account for veteran characteristics showed that veterans with a head injury had higher PTSD and depression symptom scores. Additionally, veterans with a head injury were more likely to use the health care system and to face challenges with access and continuity of care.

Interviews with veterans with TBI and caregivers of veterans with TBI (Chapter Four) reflected the findings from the umbrella review and survey analysis and added an enhanced portrait of hardship and resilience that characterizes the veteran and caregiver journeys. All of the veterans we interviewed had sustained multiple brain injuries, and all experienced continued challenges related to cognition, pain, mental health, employment, and relationships. Caregivers similarly described a heavy burden of care and worries about what the future would bring. Many were surviving, and only a few were thriving in their personal and professional lives. All had to create a new normal to account for their complex injuries—TBI, and often PTSD, among them. Looking to the future, there are opportunities to improve communication and support surrounding long-term outcomes and to promote mental and physical wellness.

In Chapter Five, we presented an evidence map of interventions to treat long-term issues associated with TBI. An evidence map is useful for depicting where evidence is strong and where it is lacking—that is, where more studies are needed to more definitively show whether a treatment is effective. Evidence supported cognitive rehabilitation for cognitive outcomes, psychotherapy for psychological outcomes, behavioral interventions for social outcomes, occupational rehabilitation for occupational outcomes, and psychotherapy and behavioral interventions for PCS. Findings were mixed for the effect of heterogeneous interventions on clinically meaningful outcomes; in many systematic reviews, the authors concluded that the findings were uncertain or inconclusive or that the evidence was too weak to draw a conclusion. Furthermore, most TBI research was conducted among the general adult population rather than veteran-specific populations. Additionally, many studies mixed analyses of TBI with other non-TBI neurological diagnoses, which may result in imprecise or inaccurate efficacy of interventions to support veterans with TBI specifically. Innovations and traditional treatments for TBI show promise, but additional high-quality research examining veteran populations is essential to understanding the most-effective interventions for improving outcomes after TBI.

To understand how easy or difficult it is for veterans to access TBI treatment and resources, we conducted a systematic web and database search and identified and categorized

2,325 TBI-related resources, which we developed into a searchable tool that we used for our analysis (Chapter Six). Of these resources, about half provided physical and mental health care. About one-fourth provided services specifically for veterans with TBI. To estimate veterans' access to TBI resources, we mapped the driving difference between the zip code of each TBI resource in the database and the zip codes of veterans who were engaged with WWP. (As noted elsewhere in this report, WWP alumni are not necessarily representative of the overall post-9/11 veteran population.) We found that most WWP alumni lived within a 60-minute drive of a VA medical center and had, on average, two veteran-specific TBI resources available to them within a 60-minute drive. WWP alumni with self-reported TBI had somewhat better geographic access to TBI resources than those without TBI did.

Finally, we presented qualitative findings from semi-structured interviews with subject-matter experts who research or treat TBI (Chapter Seven). Experts diverged on whether there is an impending "tsunami" of challenges related to accelerated aging for veterans with TBI. However, all agreed that, without improvements to data collection, management, and integration, the ambiguity surrounding risk for serious health conditions, such as Alzheimer's disease, and additional challenges related to accelerated aging will persist. These improvements require significant investments in infrastructural changes that would enable data integration and enhanced brain banks. But experts also cautioned that, while efforts to bolster data infrastructure, emerging technologies, and brain banks are promoted, the field cannot lose sight of the necessity to promote basic tenets of health and wellness for those who have sustained a TBI. Clinicians emphasized a more hopeful prognosis for those with mild TBI who are able to maintain preventive health (e.g., eating a healthy diet, exercising, following a solid sleep regimen, refraining from alcohol and substance use, and addressing mental health issues). Clinicians and researchers noted that, for those with moderate to severe TBI, consistent and proactive treatment follow-up and case management can have a significant effect on long-term prognosis.

Conclusions

Military-Related Traumatic Brain Injury Is Complex

TBI in the general adult population encompasses a complex spectrum of conditions with varying degrees of short-term and long-term consequences. The context of military service, including combat injuries and trauma, often adds challenges to the short-term and long-term healing and prognosis of a TBI.

To consider TBI as an isolated condition misses the full picture of challenges associated with military-related TBI. This especially applies to TBIs incurred in combat, which seldom happen without other serious physical injuries. In addition, the combat-related events that cause a TBI can also often lead to PTSD. More than 90 percent of WWP alumni who self-reported having a head injury on the Annual Warrior Survey also reported having PTSD. As we learned in the interviews, a veteran in a combat zone can sustain multiple TBIs that go unaddressed until the person is exposed to a major blast. In the long run, the combination of polytraumas can affect or reinforce each other. For example, both migraine pain following a TBI and PTSD-induced nightmares can greatly affect a veteran's sleep hygiene, in turn compromising cognitive abilities and increasing irritability levels. A veteran may turn to alcohol or cannabis to dull the physical and emotional pain, which may further affect relationships and the ability to engage in basic wellness. In short, a veteran's long-term health and well-being should seldom be seen as the result of one TBI and more likely as the result of multiple TBIs co-occurring with a burden of additional physical and mental health issues. With that, claims that TBI causes the early onset of neurodegenerative disorders without strictly controlling for the complex collection of additional health conditions should be interpreted with caution.

Veteran-Specific Resources Are Essential

Given the complexity of military-related TBI, treatment and resources that are targeted to the needs of veterans are critical. Providing care that is in tune with the needs of veterans also requires responsiveness to veteran- and caregiver-specific barriers to accessing care. For example, several veterans in our interview sample resided in rural regions or expressed the desire to relocate to a rural region. Our mapping analysis of TBI resources and access to care for TBI showed that WWP alumni generally had access to some TBI resources, but there was variation in the type of resource and how far away they were. Services that were more specifically tailored to TBI (e.g., VA medical centers) tended to be located farther from where veterans lived, especially for veterans living in less-populated areas of the country, where access to health care in general is more difficult.

Veterans with Traumatic Brain Injury Are Likely to Face Increasing Challenges as They Age

Although not all veterans who experience a TBI will face CTE or dementia, concerns remain for long-term effects as these veterans age. TBI results in serious long-term physical, psychological, functional, cognitive, and occupational deficits that become more complex with age and comorbidities. Functional limitations from TBI can be compounded over time and require intensive support from caregivers. Our interviews revealed that cognitive limitations were exhausting and frustrating for veterans and caregivers. Much of this caregiving falls to unpaid family members, who often support their loved ones for years and sometimes decades. Caregivers in our interviews understood that, whether or not TBI is linked to CTE or dementia, consistent, chronic care at home will be essential and likely will become more intensive as veterans age. This caregiver burden is in addition to the caregivers' own compounding age, health, and stress. Caregivers require psychological and practical support, and those needs are likely to only increase as time goes on.

In addition, veterans, especially veterans of special operations forces, were dealing with the hardship of identity loss. The journey of going from being an elite warfighter to being medically discharged and in need of care to perform daily functions was taking its toll on veterans, their caregivers, and their families. Veterans who were striving to create a new normal by seeking employment and educational opportunities also described the need for additional accommodations (e.g., needing additional time to take exams), but, in many cases, these accommodations were not granted, and veterans had to drop out of these opportunities. For some, this further compounded the mental and emotional hardship experienced when going from an active service member to a wounded veteran.

As noted earlier, clinicians emphasized that recovery from TBI requires consistent health maintenance, including a healthy diet, exercise, solid sleep hygiene, abstinence from alcohol and substance use, and treatment for any unresolved mental health issues. Hence, recovery from TBI requires attention and commitment to fundamental healthy practices.

Despite Advances in Research, Evidence of the Effects of Brain Injury Is Poor, and Research in Some Areas Is Limited

Over the past two decades, there has been an incredible investment in research on TBI. For example, since 2001, DoD has spent more than $2 billion on TBI research (U.S. House of Representatives, 2020), which has resulted in major advances in understanding and detecting brain injuries and the development of new treatment approaches. However, data on the long-term outcomes for veterans with TBI remain poor. There are few longitudinal analyses of veterans with TBI, and the majority of research focuses on outcomes from TBI in the short term (within a few years of injury). It will likely be another five to ten years before DoD and VA have an integrated electronic health record, which will allow researchers to systematically study the trajectory of care for military-related TBI as individuals move from the Military Health System to VA.

Among the research examining the long-term outcomes from TBI, very little has focused on veterans. For example, much of the research on mild TBI has been conducted in populations of athletes, which are poor proxies for the mechanisms of military-related TBI and the demographic characteristics and common comorbidities in populations of veterans.

Our analysis identified gaps in research on long-term functional, occupational, and social outcomes. These outcomes are likely very important for those with TBI, especially when considering the impact of TBI on their daily lives moving forward. In addition, most systematic reviews report on findings that are less than five years post-injury. Although such findings highlight TBI's potential lasting changes on interpersonal, societal, cognitive, and emotional functioning and biological outcomes, there are very few studies that show what these changes look like over the next ten, 20, or even 30 years. Thus, long-term investigation of TBI outcomes specifically among veterans still has a long way to go and should be a focus of future research.

Recommendations

Our findings point to several recommendations for improving care and support for veterans with TBI. These recommendations are intended to guide policymakers, health care systems, veteran-serving organizations, and researchers in their work to improve the long-term outcomes for veterans with TBI and to provide adequate support to their caregivers and families.

Create Long-Term Systems of Support

Provide Support to Veterans and Caregivers for Long-Term Planning and Expectation-Setting

The narrative accounts of veterans with TBI who participated in this study revealed the challenges of enduring a TBI (or multiple TBIs), especially for those who were injured early in the post-9/11 conflicts, when they may not have received timely or accurate diagnosis and treatment. These challenges have left veterans and caregivers with many unanswered questions about what they can expect as veterans age. Many veterans are suffering with the long-term impacts of several health issues incurred through their service, including pain, PTSD, and additional physical injuries. Veterans and caregivers need to know what they can expect in the long run and what agency they have in improving their situations, but getting those answers is complicated by the uncertainties about the long-term impacts of TBI. These circumstances underscore the importance of consistent case management. In short, veterans and their caregivers should have support so they can plan for the long term and set expectations for managing TBI and complex polytraumas.

Increase Caregiver Support

Formal long-term options for care are incomplete, and a large portion of the required support for veterans with TBI is often left to their informal family caregivers. Although family caregivers often fill gaps in support, they also age alongside their loved ones and experience their own cumulative psychological and physical burdens. These burdens on veterans and their families may be even more pronounced for veterans who suffered a TBI early in the post-9/11 conflicts, as noted earlier. For those veterans, complications may remain intensive and complex to the present day. VA's Program of Comprehensive Assistance for Family Caregivers provides support to caregivers of eligible veterans, but as our interviews with caregivers showed, more needs to be done to spread the word about the availability of this program and to reduce barriers to receiving support. In addition, as caregivers themselves age and have reduced capacity to care for their veterans, this VA program may need additional resources and an expanded mission.

Expand Access to Long-Term Care

VA does not currently pay for room and board in assisted-living facilities; however, given the expected long-term care needs of veterans with TBI, this policy may need to be reconsidered. From 2009 to 2018, VA conducted a pilot program, Assisted Living for Veterans with TBI, in which veterans with moderate to severe TBI needing long-term neurobehavioral rehabilitation were placed in private-sector TBI rehabilitation facilities (Bagalman, 2015). In its evaluation of the program submitted to the House and Senate Committees on Veterans' Affairs, VA found that the veterans in the program experienced improvements in physical and emotional health, TBI symptoms, and other outcomes, and veterans and family members were highly satisfied with the care received (VA, 2018). Currently, VA facilitates such care through the Traumatic Brain Injury – Residential Rehabilitation program but does not pay the full cost. Veterans must pay for room and board, which can be a considerable out-of-pocket expense, often $800–$1,200 per month (VA, 2018). It is critical to address the financial barriers that veterans with TBI face when long-term care is needed. VA may need additional regulatory authority to pay the full cost of long-term rehabilitation, or veterans needing such care may be warranted a supplementary disability benefit to help pay for these costs.

Expand Access to Multidisciplinary Treatment

Considering the co-occurrence of TBI and PTSD, co-locating TBI and PTSD care and research may better serve populations of veterans by delivering culturally appropriate, holistic care. To that end, expanding awareness of the existing programs and care models that provide integrated treatment of these conditions should be prioritized.

There are many treatments in use to improve outcomes in individuals with TBI, but many of these treatments are targeted to reduce problems in specific areas, even though individuals with TBI may experience deficits in multiple heterogeneous outcomes. For this reason, expanding access to tailored, multifaceted, and comprehensive treatment is important. State-of-the-art treatment centers exist, but they are few in number, geographically limited, and not positioned to take on the magnitude of military and veteran populations with complex TBI. Expanding access to this type of resource, either through technology or by widely disseminating best practices of this model, could have a high impact on veterans' quality of life and functional outcomes by delivering evidence-based TBI care that is tailored to the unique needs of veterans. Increasing the use of telehealth by revising regulations that prohibit non-VA providers to practice across state lines is a critical first step. In response to the COVID-19 pandemic, many of these regulations have been temporarily changed (Health Resources and Services Administration, 2021); making these changes permanent could improve access to care for veterans with TBI.

Promote Health-Enhancing Behaviors

As mentioned earlier, veterans and caregivers expressed frustration with the uncertainty of their long-term outcomes, and they feared early-onset dementia and other poor outcomes. The clinicians we interviewed emphasized that dementia is in no way a foregone conclusion and that veterans should be encouraged to focus on their physical health, mental health, and wellness. Our analysis of the treatment evidence showed strong support for the effect of exercise and appropriate rest on several types of outcomes. Health care providers should encourage fundamental wellness—a healthy diet, regular exercise, mindfulness, and abstinence from alcohol and other substances—as a key part of treatment. Many veteran-serving organizations already have physical fitness and health promotion as a key part of their mission; encouraging veterans with TBI to participate in these activities should be prioritized. Participation in health-promoting activities could also serve a critical social function for veterans with TBI and their caregivers, given the importance of forming personal connections to other veterans and families who understand their challenges and with whom they can share a common bond.

Collect and Integrate Better-Quality Data

Integrate Data on Traumatic Brain Injury and Related Conditions Across Record Systems

While waiting for the integrated DoD and VA electronic health record to come online, individual-level health, health care, and service history data from DoD and VA could be merged to allow for a longitudinal analysis of veterans with TBI. This type of analysis could provide, among other things, new insights into the relationships among the timing of TBI diagnosis and treatment, the types of treatment received, and long-term outcomes. A study of this type could be included as part of ongoing DoD and VA research initiatives, such as the 15-year studies that the Traumatic Brain Injury Center of Excellence is conducting.

For veterans and caregivers, better data-sharing between VA and community-based care providers would ensure better coordination of care. Veterans and caregivers expressed frustration with their perception that health care systems serving service members and veterans "don't talk to each other." This frustration was echoed by clinicians seeking medical history information on veterans and by epidemiologists who were concerned that poor tracking of TBI incidences may skew risk estimates for related conditions and other outcomes.

Enhance the WWP Annual Warrior Survey

WWP's Annual Warrior Survey is a rich source of information about the well-being of WWP alumni. To enhance the utility of this survey for informing WWP programming, advocacy, and state and federal policy recommendations, WWP should consider creating a longitudinal data file across survey years to track veterans over time. WWP may also consider additional surveys among subpopulations identified in the Annual Warrior Survey, including alumni with a head injury. The goals of these surveys would be to collect more-detailed and tailored information about barriers and challenges that alumni face in accessing health, education, employment, and even WWP programs and services.

Invest in Research

Our findings indicate a high demand and necessity for high-quality research examining veterans with TBI and corresponding treatments and outcomes. Several treatments, including those facilitated by technology and virtual care, show promise for improving outcomes associated with TBI, but there is not yet sufficient evidence for widespread application, especially in veteran populations. Expanding telehealth interventions and their rigorous evaluation could be an important means of closing gaps in veterans' access to care, particularly for veterans living in rural regions and those who are not able to reach TBI-specific treatment centers.

Conduct Longitudinal Studies Examining Variation in Outcomes and Across Different Populations

Most systematic reviews in our study focused on outcomes among the general adult population; only one-third of the reviews focused on veterans. Veterans with TBI differ in important ways from the general adult population; the cause of injury is one of the most important differences, especially when the TBI is combat-related. We also found that only a few systematic reviews examined differences in outcomes by race or gender, which is a major oversight, given the expanding diversity of the post-9/11 veteran population. A better understanding of the long-term outcomes for veterans with TBI—as well as the intersection among veteran status, race, and gender and how it contributes to access to treatment and outcomes—is critical to improving care for this most diverse population of veterans in the history of the military.

Conduct Studies on Evidence-Based Treatments, Including Holistic Treatments, for Traumatic Brain Injury

The complexity of TBI and its pervasive, lasting, and differing effects contribute to the gaps in literature on treating TBI. Current treatments are likely to be intensive, time-consuming, and expensive, which can limit the accessibility and usability of treatment. This gap in treatment research may improve when the longer-term effects of TBI are better understood and a greater variety of treatment options are available, including promising treatments that can be used at home or through technology.

Of note, although hyperbaric oxygen therapy is often considered in TBI treatment, VA and DoD clinical practice guidelines recommend against it for mild TBI (VA and DoD, 2021), and the U.S. Food and Drug Administration has not approved the therapy for treating TBI (U.S. Food and Drug Administration, 2013, 2021). Evidence for hyperbaric oxygen therapy is incomplete: Most research has focused on its use in inpatient settings for veterans with severe TBI during the acute phase of injury, and the little evidence across studies in cognitive, psychological, and mild TBI outcomes does not support its use for treatment of long-term problems from TBI.

Expand Basic Science Research

In our interviews, researchers underscored the advantages that would be conveyed to the field of TBI studies if there were reliable biomarkers for TBI severity and CTE. Although efforts in this space are well underway, advancing this research could make a significant contribution to *in vivo* diagnostics and more-timely treatment. In the meantime, brain banks are making advancements in the underlying pathology of TBI and its impacts on the brain. To that aim, veterans could be made more aware of tissue-donation options.

Closing Thoughts

WWP, DoD, VA, veterans, and caregivers have all raised concerns about the long-term consequences of military-related TBI. In particular, they are concerned about the risk for early-onset neurodegenerative disorders in an already vulnerable population.

These concerns are not unfounded, but the magnitude of the risk may not be as dire as it is sometimes portrayed to be. That being said, TBI has varying degrees of severity. Those with a mild TBI may see their symptoms resolve in a matter of weeks. Unfortunately, those with more-severe TBI may be at a higher risk for adverse long-term outcomes. Compounding this risk is the fact that severe TBI stemming from a military context often co-occurs with other serious physical, physiological, and mental health conditions.

Asking what *will* happen to veterans with TBI can turn attention away from the fact that veterans with complex polytraumas, TBI among them, have been experiencing challenges for years. For them, the problems of here and now deserve attention, support, and resources to help them, their caregivers, and their families with daily life. And, of course, these veterans and their caregivers are aging, and their challenges may only intensify in the years and decades to come.

The recommendations put forth in this report could go a long way toward ensuring that veterans who served and made significant sacrifices for the United States do not fall through the cracks. Implementing these recommendations will require a collaborative approach among veteran-serving organizations, VA, DoD, and other federal and state-level policymakers to ensure that veterans with TBI receive evidence-based treatments and interventions over the long term, along with support and resources for them and their caregivers as they age.

Search Terms for the Umbrella Review of the Risk or Prevalence of Long-Term Outcomes Following Traumatic Brain Injury

Database	Search Terms
PubMed	("Brain Injuries/complications"[MAJR] OR "Brain Injuries, Traumatic"[Mesh] OR tbi[tiab] OR traumatic brain injur*[tiab] OR mtbi[tiab] OR "brain concussion" [Mesh] OR concussion[tiab] OR concussed[tiab] OR concussive[tiab] OR head injur*[tiab]) AND ("Long term"[tiab] OR risk factor*[tiab] OR association[tiab] OR ((((deploy*[tiab] AND return*[tiab]) OR post-deployment[tiab])) AND diagnos*[tiab])) Limits: Systematic Review; Meta Analysis OR ("Brain Injuries/complications"[MAJR] OR "Brain Injuries, Traumatic"[Mesh] OR tbi[tiab] OR traumatic brain injur*[tiab] OR mtbi[tiab] OR "brain concussion" [Mesh] OR concussion[tiab] OR concussed[tiab] OR concussive[tiab]) AND ("Long term"[tiab] OR risk factor*[tiab] OR association[tiab] OR ((((deploy*[tiab] AND return*[tiab]) OR post-deployment[tiab])) AND diagnos*[tiab])) AND "systematic review"[ti] OR "meta analysis"[ti] OR "meta analyses"[ti] OR metaanalysis[ti] OR metaanalyses[ti]
APA PsycInfo (EBSCO platform)	TI(tbi OR traumatic brain injur* OR mtbi OR concussion OR concussed OR concussive) OR AB(tbi OR traumatic brain injur* OR mtbi OR concussion OR concussed OR concussive OR "head injur*") OR DE "Traumatic Brain Injury" OR DE "brain concussion" AND TI("Long term") OR "risk factor*" OR association OR (((TI(deploy* AND return*) OR TI(post-deployment))) AND TI(diagnos*)) OR AB("Long term") OR "risk factor*" OR association OR (((AB(deploy* AND return*) OR AB(post-deployment))) AND AB(diagnos*)) OR (((AB(deploy* AND return*) OR AB(post-deployment))) AND TI(diagnos*)) OR (((TI(deploy* AND return*) OR TI(post-deployment))) AND AB(diagnos*)) AND TI("systematic review" OR "meta analysis" OR "meta analyses" OR metaanalysis OR metaanalyses) OR MR("systematic review" OR "meta analysis")

Database	Search Terms
Web of Science	TS=(tbi OR traumatic brain injur* OR mtbi OR concussion OR concussed OR concussive OR head injur*) AND TS=("long term" OR "risk factor*" OR association) OR (TS=(deploy AND return) OR (TS=(post-deployment)) AND TS=(diagnos*)) AND TI=(systematic review) OR TI=(meta analysis) OR TI=(meta analyses) OR TI=(metaanalysis) OR TI=(metaanalyses)
PROSPERO	(tbi OR traumatic brain injur* OR mtbi OR concussion OR concussed OR concussive OR head injur*) AND (Systematic Review OR Meta-Analysis):RT AND (long term OR risk factor* OR association):TI,KW,RQ,SM AND (Systematic Review OR Meta-Analysis):RT

Additional Analyses of WWP Survey Data

We analyzed aggregated data from the 2017, 2018, and 2020 cross-sectional Annual Warrior Surveys. Tables B.1–B.3 of this appendix supplement the results from our analyses of WWP alumni with TBI and other head injuries (see Chapter Three).

TABLE B.1

WWP Survey Response Rate, by Year

Year	Response	Non-Response	Response Rate (%)	Total
2017	34,822	58,031	37.5	92,853
2018	33,067	64,987	33.7	98,054
2020	28,282	93,699	23.2	121,981
All	96,171	216,717	30.7	312,888

TABLE B.2

Predictors of Self-Reported Health

Predictor	Bivariate (Unadjusted)		Adjusted	
	β	*p*-Value	β	*p*-Value
Veteran has head injury	−0.24	< 0.0001	0.04	< 0.0001
Total number of physical injuries	-0.09	< 0.0001	−0.04	< 0.0001
Total number of mental injuries	−0.21	< 0.0001	−0.13	< 0.0001
Total number of activities requiring assistance	−0.11	< 0.0001	−0.08	< 0.0001
Total number of WWP programs that the veteran participates in	−0.02	< 0.0001	0.02	< 0.0001
Hazardous drinking	0.03	< 0.0001	0.00	0.9417
Drug use	−0.17	< 0.0001	−0.03	< 0.0001
Age				
18–30 (reference)				
31–45	−0.14	< 0.0001	−0.08	< 0.0001
46–60	−0.27	< 0.0001	−0.20	< 0.0001
61+	−0.19	< 0.0001	−0.18	< 0.0001
Gender				
Men (reference)				
Women	0.00	0.8798	−0.03	< 0.0001
Educational attainment				
< High school diploma, high school diploma, or GED diploma (reference)				
Some college, business, or vocational school	−0.01	0.2035	0.02	0.0292
Associate's or bachelor's degree	0.10	< 0.0001	0.09	< 0.0001
More than a college degree	0.22	< 0.0001	0.17	< 0.0001
Race/ethnicity				
White, non-Hispanic (reference)				
Black, non-Hispanic	−0.12	< 0.0001	−0.06	< 0.0001
Hispanic	−0.14	< 0.0001	−0.05	< 0.0001
American Indian or Alaska Native	−0.19	< 0.0001	−0.04	0.0008
Asian	−0.12	< 0.0001	−0.11	< 0.0001
Native Hawaiian	−0.26	< 0.0001	−0.09	< 0.0001
Other	−0.21	< 0.0001	−0.06	0.0007

Table B.2—Continued

Predictor	Bivariate (Unadjusted)		Adjusted	
	β	p-Value	β	p-Value
Marital status				
Married (reference)				
Widowed	−0.05	0.2188	0.00	0.9067
Divorced	−0.04	< 0.0001	−0.03	< 0.0001
Separated	−0.09	< 0.0001	−0.04	0.0095
Single	0.09	< 0.0001	−0.02	0.0075
Housing status				
Live in military housing (reference)				
Rent or own my own home	−0.28	< 0.0001	−0.10	< 0.0001
Share a dwelling	−0.33	< 0.0001	−0.14	< 0.0001
Live alone	−0.31	< 0.0001	−0.14	0.0059
Transitional or Section 8 housing	−0.50	< 0.0001	−0.24	< 0.0001
Supported housing, assisted-living facility, or nursing home	−0.46	< 0.0001	−0.17	0.0007
Homeless or in a shelter	−0.64	< 0.0001	−0.31	< 0.0001

TABLE B.3

Predictors of Sleep Quality

Predictor	Bivariate (Unadjusted)		Adjusted	
	β	p-Value	β	p-Value
Veteran has head injury	1.44	< 0.0001	0.09	0.0848
Total number of physical injuries	0.41	< 0.0001	0.15	< 0.0001
Total number of mental injuries	1.28	< 0.0001	0.97	< 0.0001
Total number of activities requiring assistance	0.44	< 0.0001	0.27	< 0.0001
Total number of WWP programs that the veteran participates in	0.24	< 0.0001	0.01	0.3728
Hazardous drinking	0.57	< 0.0001	0.47	< 0.0001
Drug use	1.38	< 0.0001	0.42	< 0.0001
Age				
18–30 (reference)				
31–45	0.81	< 0.0001	0.29	0.0069
46–60	0.86	< 0.0001	0.43	0.0001
61+	−0.09	0.6118	0.02	0.9152
Gender				
Men (reference)				
Women	0.54	< 0.0001	0.49	< 0.0001
Educational attainment				
< High school diploma, high school diploma, or GED diploma (reference)				
Some college, business, or vocational school	0.26	0.0101	−0.09	0.3416
Associate's or bachelor's degree	−0.13	0.196	−0.24	0.0113
More than a college degree	−0.71	< 0.0001	−0.38	0.0004
Race/ethnicity				
White, non-Hispanic (reference)				
Black, non-Hispanic	0.77	< 0.0001	0.40	< 0.0001
Hispanic	0.61	< 0.0001	0.09	0.1744
American Indian or Alaska Native	0.97	< 0.0001	0.09	0.4375
Asian	0.29	0.0481	0.43	0.0024
Native Hawaiian	0.86	< 0.0001	−0.03	0.8868
Other	0.59	0.0047	−0.12	0.5332

Table B.3—Continued

Predictor	Bivariate (Unadjusted)		Adjusted	
	β	p-Value	β	p-Value
Marital status				
Married (reference)				
Widowed	−0.04	0.9156	−0.29	0.4127
Divorced	0.63	< 0.0001	0.36	< 0.0001
Separated	0.71	< 0.0001	0.23	0.0872
Single	−0.13	0.1365	0.20	0.0294
Housing status				
Live in military housing (reference)				
Rent or own my own home	0.86	< 0.0001	−0.05	0.7925
Share a dwelling	1.10	< 0.0001	−0.08	0.7096
Live alone	1.69	< 0.0001	0.60	0.2592
Transitional or Section 8 housing	1.72	0.0032	0.27	0.4205
Supported housing, assisted-living facility, or nursing home	1.12	< 0.0001	−0.26	0.5335
Homeless or living in a shelter	2.37	0.0109	0.45	0.3372

Search Terms for the Umbrella Review of Traumatic Brain Injury Treatments and Interventions

Database	Search Terms
PubMed	"Brain Injuries/complications"[MAJR] OR "Brain Injuries, Traumatic"[Mesh] OR tbi[tiab] OR traumatic brain injur*[tiab] OR mtbi[tiab] OR "brain concussion" [Mesh] OR concussion[tiab] OR concussed[tiab] OR concussive[tiab] AND intervention*[tiab] OR treatment*[tiab] Limits: Systematic Review; Meta Analysis OR "Brain Injuries/complications"[MAJR] OR "Brain Injuries, Traumatic"[Mesh] OR tbi[tiab] OR traumatic brain injur*[tiab] OR mtbi[tiab] OR "brain concussion" [Mesh] OR concussion[tiab] OR concussed[tiab] OR concussive[tiab] AND intervention*[tiab] OR treatment*[tiab] AND "systematic review"[ti] OR "meta analysis"[ti] OR "meta analyses"[ti] OR metaanalysis[ti] OR metaanalyses[ti]
APA PsycInfo (EBSCO platform)	TI(tbi OR traumatic brain injur* OR mtbi OR concussion OR concussed OR concussive) OR AB(tbi OR traumatic brain injur* OR mtbi OR concussion OR concussed OR concussive) OR DE "Traumatic Brain Injury" OR DE "brain concussion" AND TI (intervention* OR treatment*) OR AB(intervention* OR treatment*) AND TI("systematic review" OR "meta analysis" OR "meta analyses" OR metaanalysis OR metaanalyses) OR MR("systematic review" OR "meta analysis")
Web of Science	TS=(tbi OR traumatic brain injur* OR mtbi OR concussion OR concussed OR concussive) AND TS=(intervention* OR treatment*) AND TI=("systematic review" OR "meta analysis" OR "meta analyses" OR metaanalysis OR metaanalyses)
PROSPERO	(tbi OR traumatic brain injur* OR mtbi OR concussion OR concussed OR concussive) AND (Systematic Review OR Meta-Analysis):RT AND (intervention* OR treatment*):TI,KW,RQ,SM AND (Systematic Review OR Meta-Analysis):RT

Additional Analyses of Traumatic Brain Injury Resources

This appendix supplements the analyses described in Chapter Six stemming from the database of TBI resources that we built.

We found that, on average, there were 0.97 (SD = 2.03) hospitals within a 30-minute drive of WWP alumni (using the address for hospitals in our database and the centroid of the veteran's home zip code) and that the number rose to 2.44 (SD = 3.67) hospitals when the drive time was extended to 60 minutes. Figure D.1 is a heat map that shows the geographic accessibility of hospitals within a 60-minute drive of veterans' zip codes. The darker the shading,

FIGURE D.1
Hospitals Within a 60-Minute Drive of WWP Alumni

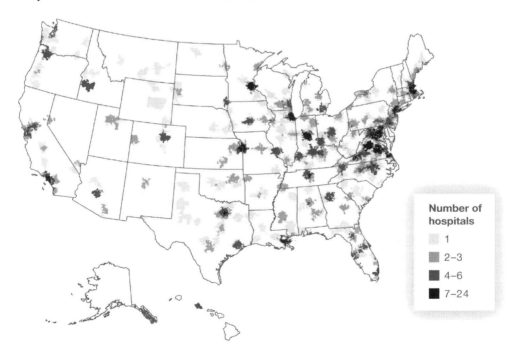

Number of hospitals
- 1
- 2–3
- 4–6
- 7–24

NOTE: White spaces are all census tracts where there are no hospitals within a 60-minute drive.

the more hospitals that are within the drive time. The numbers were slightly larger for zip codes where WWP alumni with TBI lived for both the 30-minute (mean = 1.06, SD = 2.05) and 60-minute (mean = 2.69, SD = 3.76) drive times. The results imply that WWP alumni in general and those with a TBI had access to at least one hospital within a 30-minute or 60-minute drive.

We generally found that veterans had less access to TBI resources offering mental health care than to those offering physical health care. For example, for zip codes where a WWP alumnus lived, the average number of TBI resources offering mental health care within a 30-minute drive (mean = 1.94, SD = 3.82) and a 60-minute drive (mean = 5.12, SD = 7.44) was less than the average number of resources offering physical health care for the same drive times (30-minute mean = 2.04, SD = 4.11; 60-minute mean = 5.31, SD = 8.03). Figures D.2 and D.3 show the geographic accessibility to mental and physical health care, respectively, within a 60-minute drive. We found greater access for zip codes where WWP alumni with self-reported TBI lived. In those cases, we found that the average number of TBI resources offering mental health care was 2.17 (SD = 3.97) within a 30-minute drive and 5.68 (SD = 7.59) within a 60-minute drive. Similar increases in geographic access were found for TBI resources

FIGURE D.2

Traumatic Brain Injury Resources Offering Mental Health Care Within a 60-Minute Drive of WWP Alumni

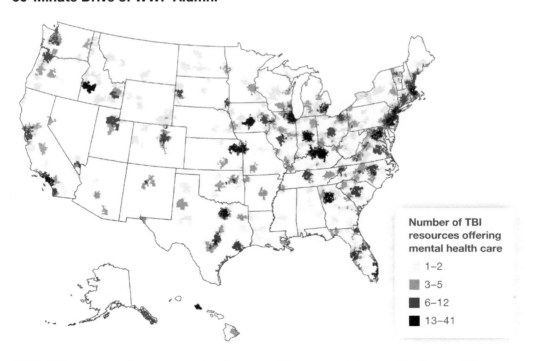

NOTE: White spaces are all census tracts where there are no TBI resources offering mental health care within a 60-minute drive.

FIGURE D.3

Traumatic Brain Injury Resources Offering Physical Health Care Within a 60-Minute Drive of WWP Alumni

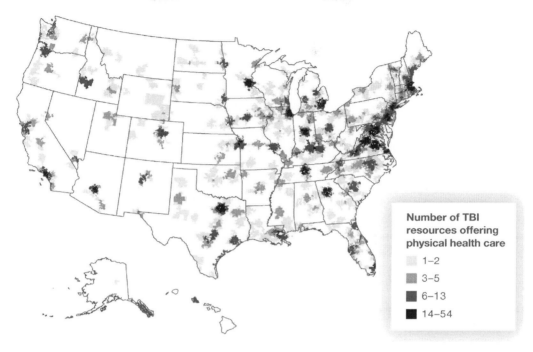

Number of TBI
resources offering
physical health care

- 1–2
- 3–5
- 6–13
- 14–54

NOTE: White spaces are all census tracts where there are no TBI resources offering physical health care within a 60-minute drive.

offering physical health care when we examined zip codes where a WWP alumnus with self-reported TBI lived.

We also calculated the number of TBI resources offering physical therapy within both drive times. For the zip codes where any WWP alumni lived, there were, on average, 0.76 (SD = 1.76) physical therapy programs within a 30-minute drive and 2.03 (SD = 3.55) such programs within a 60-minute drive. We found similar results when focusing on zip codes where a veteran with self-reported TBI lived. In those zip codes, we found that, on average, there were 0.80 (SD = 1.76) programs within a 30-minute drive and 2.15 (SD = 3.49) programs within a 60-minute drive.

We also calculated the number of resources offering occupational therapy, speech therapy, or relationship support services. We found that, within a 30-minute drive of a zip code with any WWP alumni present, relationship support services were most common (mean = 0.79, SD = 1.88), followed by speech therapy (mean = 0.73, SD = 1.73) and occupational therapy (mean = 0.71, SD = 1.71). We found the same pattern when examining resources within a 60-minute drive; that is, relationship support services were most common (mean = 2.15,

SD = 3.93), followed by speech therapy (mean = 1.96, SD = 3.49) and occupational therapy (mean = 1.93, SD = 3.49). The results for the three types of TBI resources were similar in magnitude for WWP alumni with self-reported TBI.

Abbreviations

9/11	September 11, 2001
ALS	amyotrophic lateral sclerosis
COVID-19	coronavirus disease 2019
CTE	chronic traumatic encephalopathy
DoD	U.S. Department of Defense
ER	emergency room
GED	Tests of General Educational Development
IED	improvised explosive device
OR	odds ratio
PCS	post-concussion syndrome
PICOTSS	participants, interventions, comparators, outcomes, timing, settings, and study design
PTSD	posttraumatic stress disorder
SD	standard deviation
TBI	traumatic brain injury
VA	U.S. Department of Veterans Affairs
VHA	Veterans Health Administration
WWP	Wounded Warrior Project

References

Acabchuk, R. L., J. M. Brisson, C. L. Park, N. Babbott-Bryan, O. A. Parmelee, and B. T. Johnson, "Therapeutic Effects of Meditation, Yoga, and Mindfulness-Based Interventions for Chronic Symptoms of Mild Traumatic Brain Injury: A Systematic Review and Meta-Analysis," *Applied Psychology, Health, and Well-Being*, Vol. 13, No. 1, February 2021, pp. 34–62.

Ackland, P. E., N. Greer, N. A. Sayer, M. R. Spoont, B. C. Taylor, R. MacDonald, L. McKenzie, C. Rosebush, and T. J. Wilt, "Effectiveness and Harms of Mental Health Treatments in Service Members and Veterans with Deployment-Related Mild Traumatic Brain Injury," *Journal of Affective Disorders*, Vol. 252, June 1, 2019, pp. 493–501.

Adams, Rachel Sayko, John D. Corrigan, and Mary Jo Larson, "Alcohol Use After Combat-Acquired Traumatic Brain Injury: What We Know and Don't Know," *Journal of Social Work Practice in the Addictions*, Vol. 12, No. 1, 2012, pp. 28–51.

Ahorsu, D. K., E. S. Adjaottor, and B. Y. H. Lam, "Intervention Effect of Non-Invasive Brain Stimulation on Cognitive Functions Among People with Traumatic Brain Injury: A Systematic Review and Meta-Analysis," *Brain Sciences*, Vol. 11, No. 7, June 24, 2021.

Al Sayegh, A., D. Sandford, and A. J. Carson, "Psychological Approaches to Treatment of Postconcussion Syndrome: A Systematic Review," *Journal of Neurology, Neurosurgery, and Psychiatry*, Vol. 81, No. 10, October 2010, pp. 1128–1134.

Alashram, A. R., G. Annino, E. Padua, C. Romagnoli, and N. B. Mercuri, "Cognitive Rehabilitation Post Traumatic Brain Injury: A Systematic Review for Emerging Use of Virtual Reality Technology," *Journal of Clinical Neuroscience*, Vol. 66, August 2019, pp. 209–219.

Alashram, A. R., G. Annino, M. Raju, and E. Padua, "Effects of Physical Therapy Interventions on Balance Ability in People with Traumatic Brain Injury: A Systematic Review," *NeuroRehabilitation*, Vol. 46, No. 4, 2020, pp. 455–466.

Ali, J. I., J. Viczko, and C. M. Smart, "Efficacy of Neurofeedback Interventions for Cognitive Rehabilitation Following Brain Injury: Systematic Review and Recommendations for Future Research," *Journal of the International Neuropsychological Society*, Vol. 26, No. 1, January 2020, pp. 31–46.

Andelic, N., E. I. Howe, T. Hellstrom, M. F. Sanchez, J. Lu, M. Lovstad, and C. Roe, "Disability and Quality of Life 20 Years After Traumatic Brain Injury," *Brain and Behavior*, Vol. 8, No. 7, July 2018, article e01018.

Anghinah, Renato, Robson Luís Oliveira de Amorim, Wellingson Silva Paiva, Magali Taino Schmidt, and Jéssica Natuline Ianof, "Traumatic Brain Injury Pharmacological Treatment: Recommendations," *Arquivos de Neuro-Psiquiatria*, Vol. 76, No. 2, February 2018, pp. 100–103.

Arbabi, M., R. Sheldon, P. Bahadoran, J. G. Smith, N. Poole, and N. Agrawal, "Treatment Outcomes in Mild Traumatic Brain Injury: A Systematic Review of Randomized Controlled Trials," *Brain Injury*, Vol. 34, No. 9, July 28, 2020, pp. 1139–1149.

Argyriou, A. A., D. D. Mitsikostas, E. Mantovani, P. Litsardopoulos, V. Panagiotopoulos, and S. Tamburin, "An Updated Brief Overview on Post-Traumatic Headache and a Systematic Review of the Non-Pharmacological Interventions for Its Management," *Expert Review of Neurotherapeutics*, Vol. 21, No. 4, April 2021, pp. 475–490.

Bagalman, Erin, *Health Care for Veterans: Traumatic Brain Injury*, Washington, D.C.: Congressional Research Service, R40941, March 9, 2015.

Bahraini, Nazanin H., Grahame K. Simpson, Lisa A. Brenner, Adam S. Hoffberg, and Alexandra L. Schneider, "Suicidal Ideation and Behaviours After Traumatic Brain Injury: A Systematic Review," *Brain Impairment*, Vol. 14, No. 1, 2013, pp. 92–112.

Baker, A., S. Barker, A. Sampson, and C. Martin, "Caregiver Outcomes and Interventions: A Systematic Scoping Review of the Traumatic Brain Injury and Spinal Cord Injury Literature," *Clinical Rehabilitation*, Vol. 31, No. 1, January 2017, pp. 45–60.

Ballesteros, Javier, Itziar Güemes, Nora Ibarra, and José I. Quemada, "The Effectiveness of Donepezil for Cognitive Rehabilitation After Traumatic Brain Injury: A Systematic Review," *Journal of Head Trauma Rehabilitation*, Vol. 23, No. 3, May 2008, pp. 171–180.

Barker-Collo, S., N. Starkey, and A. Theadom, "Treatment for Depression Following Mild Traumatic Brain Injury in Adults: A Meta-Analysis," *Brain Injury*, Vol. 27, No. 10, 2013, pp. 1124–1133.

Barlow, K. M., M. J. Esser, M. Veidt, and R. Boyd, "Melatonin as a Treatment After Traumatic Brain Injury: A Systematic Review and Meta-Analysis of the Pre-Clinical and Clinical Literature," *Journal of Neurotrauma*, Vol. 36, No. 4, February 15, 2019, pp. 523–537.

Bazarian, Jeffrey J., Ibolja Cernak, Linda Noble-Haeusslein, Samuel Potolicchio, and Nancy Temkin, "Long-Term Neurologic Outcomes After Traumatic Brain Injury," *Journal of Head Trauma Rehabilitation*, Vol. 24, No. 6, November–December 2009, pp. 439–451.

Beadle, Elizabeth Jane, Tamara Ownsworth, Jennifer Fleming, and David Shum, "The Impact of Traumatic Brain Injury on Self-Identity: A Systematic Review of the Evidence for Self-Concept Changes," *Journal of Head Trauma Rehabilitation*, Vol. 31, No. 2, March–April 2016, pp. E12–E25.

Beedham, W., A. Belli, S. Ingaralingam, S. Haque, and R. Upthegrove, "The Management of Depression Following Traumatic Brain Injury: A Systematic Review with Meta-Analysis," *Brain Injury*, Vol. 34, No. 10, August 23, 2020, pp. 1287–1304.

Belanger, H. G., G. Curtiss, J. A. Demery, B. K. Lebowitz, and R. D. Vanderploeg, "Factors Moderating Neuropsychological Outcomes Following Mild Traumatic Brain Injury: A Meta-Analysis," *Journal of the International Neuropsychological Society*, Vol. 11, No. 3, May 2005, pp. 215–227.

Bengtsson, M., and A. K. Godbolt, "Effects of Acetylcholinesterase Inhibitors on Cognitive Function in Patients with Chronic Traumatic Brain Injury: A Systematic Review," *Journal of Rehabilitation Medicine*, Vol. 48, No. 1, January 2016, pp. 1–5.

Berger, S., J. Kaldenberg, R. Selmane, and S. Carlo, "Effectiveness of Interventions to Address Visual and Visual-Perceptual Impairments to Improve Occupational Performance in Adults with Traumatic Brain Injury: A Systematic Review," *American Journal of Occupational Therapy*, Vol. 70, No. 3, May–June 2016.

Bergersen, K., J. Ø. Halvorsen, E. A. Tryti, S. I. Taylor, and A. Olsen, "A Systematic Literature Review of Psychotherapeutic Treatment of Prolonged Symptoms After Mild Traumatic Brain Injury," *Brain Injury*, Vol. 31, No. 3, 2017, pp. 279–289.

Betts, S., L. Feichter, Z. Kleinig, A. O'Connell-Debais, H. Thai, C. Wong, and S. Kumar, "Telerehabilitation Versus Standard Care for Improving Cognitive Function and Quality of Life for Adults with Traumatic Brain Injury: A Systematic Review," *Internet Journal of Allied Health Sciences and Practice*, Vol. 16, No. 3, 2018, article 9.

Bjork, James M., and Steven J. Grant, "Does Traumatic Brain Injury Increase Risk for Substance Abuse?" *Journal of Neurotrauma*, Vol. 26, No. 7, July 2009, pp. 1077–1082.

Bland, D. C., C. Zampieri, and D. L. Damiano, "Effectiveness of Physical Therapy for Improving Gait and Balance in Individuals with Traumatic Brain Injury: A Systematic Review," *Brain Injury*, Vol. 25, No. 7–8, 2011, pp. 664–679.

Bogdanov, S., S. Naismith, and S. Lah, "Sleep Outcomes Following Sleep-Hygiene-Related Interventions for Individuals with Traumatic Brain Injury: A Systematic Review," *Brain Injury*, Vol. 31, No. 4, 2017, pp. 422–433.

Bogdanova, Y., M. K. Yee, V. T. Ho, and K. D. Cicerone, "Computerized Cognitive Rehabilitation of Attention and Executive Function in Acquired Brain Injury: A Systematic Review," *Journal of Head Trauma Rehabilitation*, Vol. 31, No. 6, November–December 2016, pp. 419–433.

Bogner, Jennifer, and John D. Corrigan, "Interventions for Substance Misuse Following TBI: A Systematic Review," *Brain Impairment*, Vol. 14, No. 1, 2013, pp. 77–91.

Borghol, Amne, Michael Aucoin, Ifeanyichukwu Onor, Dana Jamero, and Fadi Hawawini, "Modafinil for the Improvement of Patient Outcomes Following Traumatic Brain Injury," *Innovations in Clinical Neuroscience*, Vol. 15, No. 3–4, 2018, pp. 17–23.

Boston University CTE Center, "VA-BU-CLF Brain Bank," webpage, undated. As of November 29, 2021:
https://www.bu.edu/cte/our-research/brain-bank/

Bradley, K. A., K. R. Bush, A. J. Epler, D. J. Dobie, T. M. Davis, J. L. Sporleder, C. Maynard, M. L. Burman, and D. R. Kivlahan, "Two Brief Alcohol-Screening Tests from the Alcohol Use Disorders Identification Test (AUDIT): Validation in a Female Veterans Affairs Patient Population," *Archives of Internal Medicine*, Vol. 163, No. 7, April 14, 2003, pp. 821–829.

Brain Injury Association of America, homepage, undated. As of November 1, 2021:
https://www.biausa.org

Brainline, homepage, undated. As of November 1, 2021:
https://www.brainline.org/resource-directory

Brassel, S., E. Power, A. Campbell, M. Brunner, and L. Togher, "Recommendations for the Design and Implementation of Virtual Reality for Acquired Brain Injury Rehabilitation: Systematic Review," *Journal of Medical Internet Research*, Vol. 23, No. 7, July 30, 2021, article e26344.

Brasure, M., G. J. Lamberty, N. A. Sayer, N. W. Nelson, R. MacDonald, J. Ouellette, and T. J. Wilt, "Participation After Multidisciplinary Rehabilitation for Moderate to Severe Traumatic Brain Injury in Adults: A Systematic Review," *Archives of Physical Medicine and Rehabilitation*, Vol. 94, No. 7, July 2013, pp. 1398–1420.

Bryan, C. J., and T. A. Clemans, "Repetitive Traumatic Brain Injury, Psychological Symptoms, and Suicide Risk in a Clinical Sample of Deployed Military Personnel," *JAMA Psychiatry*, Vol. 70, No. 7, July 2013, pp. 686–691.

Buckley, L., S. A. Kaye, R. P. Stork, J. E. Heinze, and J. T. Eckner, "Traumatic Brain Injury and Aggression: A Systematic Review and Future Directions Using Community Samples," *Aggression and Violent Behavior*, Vol. 37, November 2017, pp. 26–34.

Buhagiar, F., M. Fitzgerald, J. Bell, F. Allanson, and C. Pestell, "Neuromodulation for Mild Traumatic Brain Injury Rehabilitation: A Systematic Review," *Frontiers in Human Neuroscience*, Vol. 14, 2020, article 598208.

Bush, K., D. R. Kivlahan, M. B. McDonell, S. D. Fihn, and K. A. Bradley, "The AUDIT Alcohol Consumption Questions (AUDIT-C): An Effective Brief Screening Test for Problem Drinking. Ambulatory Care Quality Improvement Project (ACQUIP). Alcohol Use Disorders Identification Test," *Archives of Internal Medicine*, Vol. 158, No. 16, September 14, 1998, pp. 1789–1795.

Butler-Kisber, L., *Qualitative Inquiry: Thematic, Narrative and Arts-Informed Perspectives*, Thousand Oaks, Calif.: Sage Publications, 2010.

Buysse, D. J., C. F. Reynolds III, T. H. Monk, S. R. Berman, and D. J. Kupfer, "The Pittsburgh Sleep Quality Index: A New Instrument for Psychiatric Practice and Research," *Psychiatry Research*, Vol. 28, No. 2, May 1989, pp. 193–213.

Cancelliere, C., V. L. Kristman, J. D. Cassidy, C. A. Hincapié, P. Côté, E. Boyle, L. J. Carroll, B. M. Stålnacke, C. Nygren-de Boussard, and J. Borg, "Systematic Review of Return to Work After Mild Traumatic Brain Injury: Results of the International Collaboration on Mild Traumatic Brain Injury Prognosis," *Archives of Physical Medicine and Rehabilitation*, Vol. 95, No. 3 Supp., March 2014, pp. S201–S209.

Cano Porras, D., P. Siemonsma, R. Inzelberg, G. Zeilig, and M. Plotnik, "Advantages of Virtual Reality in the Rehabilitation of Balance and Gait: Systematic Review," *Neurology*, Vol. 90, No. 22, May 29, 2018, pp. 1017–1025.

Cantor, J. B., T. Ashman, T. Bushnik, X. Cai, L. Farrell-Carnahan, S. Gumber, T. Hart, J. Rosenthal, and M. P. Dijkers, "Systematic Review of Interventions for Fatigue After Traumatic Brain Injury: A NIDRR Traumatic Brain Injury Model Systems Study," *Journal of Head Trauma Rehabilitation*, Vol. 29, No. 6, November–December 2014, pp. 490–497.

Carlson, K., S. Kehle, L. Meis, N. Greer, R. MacDonald, I. Rutks, and T. J. Wilt, *The Assessment and Treatment of Individuals with History of Traumatic Brain Injury and Post-Traumatic Stress Disorder: A Systematic Review of the Evidence*, Washington, D.C.: U.S. Department of Veterans Affairs, August 2009.

Carney, N., R. M. Chesnut, H. Maynard, N. C. Mann, P. Patterson, and M. Helfand, "Effect of Cognitive Rehabilitation on Outcomes for Persons with Traumatic Brain Injury: A Systematic Review," *Journal of Head Trauma Rehabilitation*, Vol. 14, No. 3, June 1999, pp. 277–307.

Carroll, L. J., J. D. Cassidy, C. Cancelliere, P. Côté, C. A. Hincapié, V. L. Kristman, L. W. Holm, J. Borg, C. Nygren-de Boussard, and J. Hartvigsen, "Systematic Review of the Prognosis After Mild Traumatic Brain Injury in Adults: Cognitive, Psychiatric, and Mortality Outcomes: Results of the International Collaboration on Mild Traumatic Brain Injury Prognosis," *Archives of Physical Medicine and Rehabilitation*, Vol. 95, No. 3, Supp., March 2014, pp. S152–S173.

Carter, K. M., A. N. Pauhl, and A. D. Christie, "The Role of Active Rehabilitation in Concussion Management: A Systematic Review and Meta-Analysis," *Medicine and Science in Sports and Exercise*, Vol. 53, No. 9, September 2021, pp. 1835–1845.

Cattelani, R., M. Zettin, and P. Zoccolotti, "Rehabilitation Treatments for Adults with Behavioral and Psychosocial Disorders Following Acquired Brain Injury: A Systematic Review," *Neuropsychology Review*, Vol. 20, No. 1, March 2010, pp. 52–85.

Chang, P. F., M. F. Baxter, and J. Rissky, "Effectiveness of Interventions Within the Scope of Occupational Therapy Practice to Improve Motor Function of People with Traumatic Brain Injury: A Systematic Review," *American Journal of Occupational Therapy*, Vol. 70, No. 3, May–June 2016.

Chang, W., J. Cheng, J. J. Allaire, C. Sievert, B. Schloerke, Y. Xie, J. Allen, J. McPherson, A. Dipert, and B. Borges, "shiny: Web Application Framework for R," R package version 1.6.0, 2021. As of October 21, 2021:
https://CRAN.R-project.org/package=shiny

Chapman, J. C., and R. Diaz-Arrastia, "Military Traumatic Brain Injury: A Review," *Alzheimer's and Dementia*, Vol. 10, No. 3, Supp., June 2014, pp. S97–104.

Chee, Justin N., Carol Hawley, Judith L. Charlton, Shawn Marshall, Ian Gillespie, Sjaan Koppel, Brenda Vrkljan, Debbie Ayotte, and Mark J. Rapoport, "Risk of Motor Vehicle Collision or Driving Impairment After Traumatic Brain Injury: A Collaborative International Systematic Review and Meta-Analysis," *Journal of Head Trauma Rehabilitation*, Vol. 34, No. 1, January–February 2019, pp. E27–E38.

Cheever, K., J. McDevitt, J. Phillips, and K. Kawata, "The Role of Cervical Symptoms in Post-Concussion Management: A Systematic Review," *Sports Medicine*, Vol. 51, No. 9, 2021, pp. 1875–1891.

Chen, C. L., M. Y. Lin, M. H. Huda, and P. S. Tsai, "Effects of Cognitive Behavioral Therapy for Adults with Post-Concussion Syndrome: A Systematic Review and Meta-Analysis of Randomized Controlled Trials," *Journal of Psychosomatic Research*, Vol. 136, September 2020, article 110190.

Cheng, Y. S., P. T. Tseng, Y. C. Wu, Y. K. Tu, C. K. Wu, C. W. Hsu, W. T. Lei, D. J. Li, T. Y. Chen, B. Stubbs, A. F. Carvalho, C. S. Liang, T. C. Yeh, C. S. Chu, Y. W. Chen, P. Y. Lin, M. K. Wu, and C. K. Sun, "Therapeutic Benefits of Pharmacologic and Nonpharmacologic Treatments for Depressive Symptoms After Traumatic Brain Injury: A Systematic Review and Network Meta-Analysis," *Journal of Psychiatry and Neuroscience*, Vol. 46, No. 1, January 21, 2021, pp. E196–E207.

Chien, Y. J., Y. C. Chien, C. T. Liu, H. C. Wu, C. Y. Chang, and M. Y. Wu, "Effects of Methylphenidate on Cognitive Function in Adults with Traumatic Brain Injury: A Meta-Analysis," *Brain Sciences*, Vol. 9, No. 11, 2019, article 291.

Chong, C. S., "Management Strategies for Post-Concussion Syndrome After Mild Head Injury: A Systematic Review," *Hong Kong Journal of Occupational Therapy*, Vol. 18, No. 2, July 2008, pp. 59–67.

Chung, C. S., A. Pollock, T. Campbell, B. R. Durward, and S. Hagen, "Cognitive Rehabilitation for Executive Dysfunction in Adults with Stroke or Other Adult Non-Progressive Acquired Brain Damage," *Cochrane Database of Systematic Reviews*, Vol. 2013, No. 4, April 30, 2013, article CD008391.

Chung, P., and F. Khan, "Traumatic Brain Injury (TBI): Overview of Diagnosis and Treatment," *Journal of Neurology and Neurophysiology*, Vol. 5, No. 1, 2013, article 1000182.

Cicerone, K. D., C. Dahlberg, J. F. Malec, D. M. Langenbahn, T. Felicetti, S. Kneipp, W. Ellmo, K. Kalmar, J. T. Giacino, J. P. Harley, L. Laatsch, P. A. Morse, and J. Catanese, "Evidence-Based Cognitive Rehabilitation: Updated Review of the Literature from 1998 Through 2002," *Archives of Physical Medicine and Rehabilitation*, Vol. 86, No. 8, August 2005, pp. 1681–1692.

Cicerone, K. D., Y. Goldin, K. Ganci, A. Rosenbaum, J. V. Wethe, D. M. Langenbahn, J. F. Malec, T. F. Bergquist, K. Kingsley, D. Nagele, L. Trexler, M. Fraas, Y. Bogdanova, and J. P. Harley, "Evidence-Based Cognitive Rehabilitation: Systematic Review of the Literature from 2009 Through 2014," *Archives of Physical Medicine and Rehabilitation*, Vol. 100, No. 8, August 2019, pp. 1515–1533.

Cicerone, K. D., D. M. Langenbahn, C. Braden, J. F. Malec, K. Kalmar, M. Fraas, T. Felicetti, L. Laatsch, J. P. Harley, T. Bergquist, J. Azulay, J. Cantor, and T. Ashman, "Evidence-Based Cognitive Rehabilitation: Updated Review of the Literature from 2003 Through 2008," *Archives of Physical Medicine and Rehabilitation*, Vol. 92, No. 4, April 2011, pp. 519–530.

Clay, F. J., A. J. Hicks, H. Zaman, J. Ponsford, R. Batty, L. A. Perry, and M. Hopwood, "Prophylaxis Pharmacotherapy to Prevent the Onset of Post-Traumatic Brain Injury Depression: A Systematic Review," *Journal of Neurotrauma*, Vol. 36, No. 13, July 1, 2019, pp. 2053–2064.

Comper, P., S. M. Bisschop, N. Carnide, and A. Tricco, "A Systematic Review of Treatments for Mild Traumatic Brain Injury," *Brain Injury*, Vol. 19, No. 11, October 2005, pp. 863–880.

Corrigan, J. D., and W. J. Mysiw, "Substance Misuse Among Persons with Traumatic Brain Injury," in N. D. Zasler, D. I. Katz, R. D. Zafonte, D. B. Arciniegas, M. R. Bullock, and J. S. Kreutzer, eds., *Brain Injury Medicine: Principles and Practice*, 2nd ed., New York: Demos Medical Publishing, 2012, pp. 1315–1328.

Corrigan, J. D., T. Zheng, S. M. Pinto, J. Bogner, J. Kean, J. P. Niemeier, T. P. Guerrier, B. Haaland, and S. D. Horn, "Effect of Preexisting and Co-Occurring Comorbid Conditions on Recovery in the 5 Years After Rehabilitation for Traumatic Brain Injury," *Journal of Head Trauma Rehabilitation*, Vol. 35, No. 3, May–June 2020, pp. E288–E298.

Cullen, Nora, Josie Chundamala, Mark Bayley, and Jeffrey Jutai, "The Efficacy of Acquired Brain Injury Rehabilitation," *Brain Injury*, Vol. 21, No. 2, 2007, pp. 113–132.

Cunningham, J., S. P. Broglio, M. O'Grady, and F. Wilson, "History of Sport-Related Concussion and Long-Term Clinical Cognitive Health Outcomes in Retired Athletes: A Systematic Review," *Journal of Athletic Training*, Vol. 55, No. 2, February 2020, pp. 132–158.

Cunningham, J., S. Broglio, and F. Wilson, "Influence of Playing Rugby on Long-Term Brain Health Following Retirement: A Systematic Review and Narrative Synthesis," *BMJ Open Sport and Exercise Medicine*, Vol. 4, No. 1, 2018, article e000356.

Davidson, J. R. T., C. Crawford, J. A. Ives, and W. B. Jonas, "Homeopathic Treatments in Psychiatry: A Systematic Review of Randomized Placebo-Controlled Studies," *Journal of Clinical Psychiatry*, Vol. 72, No. 6, June 2011, pp. 795–805.

Dhaliwal, Simarjot K., Benjamin P. Meek, and Mandana M. Modirrousta, "Non-Invasive Brain Stimulation for the Treatment of Symptoms Following Traumatic Brain Injury," *Frontiers in Psychiatry*, Vol. 6, 2015.

Dikmen, Sureyya S., John D. Corrigan, Harvey S. Levin, Joan Machamer, William Stiers, and Marc G. Weisskopf, "Cognitive Outcome Following Traumatic Brain Injury," *Journal of Head Trauma Rehabilitation*, Vol. 24, No. 6, November–December 2009, pp. 430–438.

Dobscha, S. K., M. E. Clark, B. J. Morasco, M. Freeman, R. Campbell, and M. Helfand, "Systematic Review of the Literature on Pain in Patients with Polytrauma Including Traumatic Brain Injury," *Pain Medicine*, Vol. 10, No. 7, October 2009, pp. 1200–1217.

Donker-Cools, B. H., J. G. Daams, H. Wind, and M. H. Frings-Dresen, "Effective Return-to-Work Interventions After Acquired Brain Injury: A Systematic Review," *Brain Injury*, Vol. 30, No. 2, 2016, pp. 113–131.

Dougall, D., N. Poole, and N. Agrawal, "Pharmacotherapy for Chronic Cognitive Impairment in Traumatic Brain Injury," *Cochrane Database of Systematic Reviews*, No. 12, December 1, 2015, article CD009221.

Dun & Bradstreet, "Sociocultural Research Consultants: Company Profile," webpage, undated. As of August 31, 2021:
https://www.dnb.com/business-directory/company-profiles.sociocultural_research_consultants_llc.60cefa2eb6984708dfdb4d9a746e2df5.html

Dunning, D. L., B. Westgate, and A. R. Adlam, "A Meta-Analysis of Working Memory Impairments in Survivors of Moderate-to-Severe Traumatic Brain Injury," *Neuropsychology*, Vol. 30, No. 7, October 2016, pp. 811–819.

Egeto, P., S. D. Badovinac, M. G. Hutchison, T. J. Ornstein, and T. A. Schweizer, "A Systematic Review and Meta-Analysis on the Association Between Driving Ability and Neuropsychological Test Performances After Moderate to Severe Traumatic Brain Injury," *Journal of the International Neuropsychological Society*, Vol. 25, No. 8, September 2019, pp. 868–877.

Elliott, M., and F. Parente, "Efficacy of Memory Rehabilitation Therapy: A Meta-Analysis of TBI and Stroke Cognitive Rehabilitation Literature," *Brain Injury*, Vol. 28, No. 12, 2014, pp. 1610–1616.

Emelifeonwu, J. A., H. Flower, J. J. Loan, K. McGivern, and P. J. D. Andrews, "Prevalence of Anterior Pituitary Dysfunction Twelve Months or More Following Traumatic Brain Injury in Adults: A Systematic Review and Meta-Analysis," *Journal of Neurotrauma*, Vol. 37, No. 2, January 2020, pp. 217–226.

Fadyl, J. K., and K. M. McPherson, "Approaches to Vocational Rehabilitation After Traumatic Brain Injury: A Review of the Evidence," *Journal of Head Trauma Rehabilitation*, Vol. 24, No. 3, May–June 2009, pp. 195–212.

Fann, J. R., T. Hart, and K. G. Schomer, "Treatment for Depression After Traumatic Brain Injury: A Systematic Review," *Journal of Neurotrauma*, Vol. 26, No. 12, December 2009, pp. 2383–2402.

Farmer, Carrie M., Heather Krull, Thomas W. Concannon, Molly Simmons, Francesca Pillemer, Teague Ruder, Andrew M. Parker, Maulik P. Purohit, Liisa Hiatt, Benjamin Batorsky, and Kimberly A. Hepner, *Understanding Treatment of Mild Traumatic Brain Injury in the Military Health System*, Santa Monica, Calif.: RAND Corporation, RR-844-OSD, 2016. As of October 19, 2021:
https://www.rand.org/pubs/research_reports/RR844.html

Fazel, S., J. Philipson, L. Gardiner, R. Merritt, and M. Grann, "Neurological Disorders and Violence: A Systematic Review and Meta-Analysis with a Focus on Epilepsy and Traumatic Brain Injury," *Journal of Neurology*, Vol. 256, No. 10, October 2009, pp. 1591–1602.

Finch, E., A. Copley, P. Cornwell, and C. Kelly, "Systematic Review of Behavioral Interventions Targeting Social Communication Difficulties After Traumatic Brain Injury," *Archives of Physical Medicine and Rehabilitation*, Vol. 97, No. 8, August 2016, pp. 1352–1365.

Fleminger, S., D. L. Oliver, S. Lovestone, S. Rabe-Hesketh, and A. Giora, "Head Injury as a Risk Factor for Alzheimer's Disease: The Evidence 10 Years On; A Partial Replication," *Journal of Neurology, Neurosurgery and Psychiatry*, Vol. 74, No. 7, July 2003, pp. 857–862.

Fralick, M., E. Sy, A. Hassan, M. J. Burke, E. Mostofsky, and T. Karsies, "Association of Concussion with the Risk of Suicide: A Systematic Review and Meta-Analysis," *JAMA Neurology*, Vol. 76, No. 2, February 1, 2019, pp. 144–151.

Frenette, A. J., S. Kanji, L. Rees, D. R. Williamson, M. M. Perreault, A. F. Turgeon, F. Bernard, and D. A. Fergusson, "Efficacy and Safety of Dopamine Agonists in Traumatic Brain Injury: A Systematic Review of Randomized Controlled Trials," *Journal of Neurotrauma*, Vol. 29, No. 1, January 1, 2012, pp. 1–18.

Fritz, N. E., F. M. Cheek, and D. S. Nichols-Larsen, "Motor-Cognitive Dual-Task Training in Persons with Neurologic Disorders: A Systematic Review," *Journal of Neurologic Physical Therapy*, Vol. 39, No. 3, July 2015, pp. 142–153.

Frueh, B. C., A. Madan, J. C. Fowler, S. Stomberg, M. Bradshaw, K. Kelly, B. Weinstein, M. Luttrell, S. G. Danner, and D. C. Beidel, "'Operator Syndrome': A Unique Constellation of Medical and Behavioral Health-Care Needs of Military Special Operation Forces," *International Journal of Psychiatry in Medicine*, Vol. 55, No. 4, July 2020, pp. 281–295.

Gallo, V., K. Motley, S. P. T. Kemp, S. Mian, T. Patel, L. James, N. Pearce, and D. McElvenny, "Concussion and Long-Term Cognitive Impairment Among Professional or Elite Sport-Persons: A Systematic Review," *Journal of Neurology, Neurosurgery and Psychiatry*, Vol. 91, No. 5, May 2020, pp. 455–468.

Gao, C., Q. Fu, P. Chen, Z. Liu, and Q. Zhou, "The Influence of Sertraline on Depressive Disorder After Traumatic Brain Injury: A Meta-Analysis of Randomized Controlled Studies," *American Journal of Emergency Medicine*, Vol. 37, No. 9, September 2019, pp. 1778–1783.

Gardner, R. C., A. L. Byers, D. E. Barnes, Y. Li, J. Boscardin, and K. Yaffe, "Mild TBI and Risk of Parkinson Disease: A Chronic Effects of Neurotrauma Consortium Study," *Neurology*, Vol. 90, No. 20, May 15, 2018, pp. E1771–E1779.

Geraldo, Andreia, Artemisa R. Dores, Bárbara Coelho, Eduarda Ramião, Alexandre Castro-Caldas, and Fernando Barbosa, "Efficacy of ICT-Based Neurocognitive Rehabilitation Programs for Acquired Brain Injury: A Systematic Review on Its Assessment Methods," *European Psychologist*, Vol. 23, No. 3, 2018, pp. 250–264.

Gertler, P., R. L. Tate, and I. D. Cameron, "Non-Pharmacological Interventions for Depression in Adults and Children with Traumatic Brain Injury," *Cochrane Database of Systematic Reviews*, No. 12, December 14, 2015, article CD009871.

Godbolt, A. K., C. Cancelliere, C. A. Hincapié, C. Marras, E. Boyle, V. L. Kristman, V. G. Coronado, and J. D. Cassidy, "Systematic Review of the Risk of Dementia and Chronic Cognitive Impairment After Mild Traumatic Brain Injury: Results of the International Collaboration on Mild Traumatic Brain Injury Prognosis," *Archives of Physical Medicine and Rehabilitation*, Vol. 95, No. 3, Supp., March 2014, pp. S245–S256.

Gormley, M., M. Devanaboyina, N. Andelic, C. Røe, R. T. Seel, and J. Lu, "Long-Term Employment Outcomes Following Moderate to Severe Traumatic Brain Injury: A Systematic Review and Meta-Analysis," *Brain Injury*, Vol. 33, No. 13–14, 2019, pp. 1567–1580.

Greer, N., P. Ackland, N. Sayer, M. Spoont, B. Taylor, R. MacDonald, L. McKenzie, C. Rosebush, and T. J. Wilt, *Relationship of Deployment-Related Mild Traumatic Brain Injury to Posttraumatic Stress Disorder, Depressive Disorders, Substance Use Disorders, Suicidal Ideation, and Anxiety Disorders: A Systematic Review*, Washington, D.C.: U.S. Department of Veterans Affairs, March 2019.

Greer, N., N. A. Sayer, M. Spoont, B. C. Taylor, P. E. Ackland, R. MacDonald, L. McKenzie, C. Rosebush, and T. J. Wilt, "Prevalence and Severity of Psychiatric Disorders and Suicidal Behavior in Service Members and Veterans With and Without Traumatic Brain Injury: Systematic Review," *Journal of Head Trauma Rehabilitation*, Vol. 35, No. 1, January–February 2020, pp. 1–13.

Grima, N., J. Ponsford, S. M. Rajaratnam, D. Mansfield, and M. P. Pase, "Sleep Disturbances in Traumatic Brain Injury: A Meta-Analysis," *Journal of Clinical Sleep Medicine*, Vol. 12, No. 3, March 2016, pp. 419–428.

Hallock, H., D. Collins, A. Lampit, K. Deol, J. Fleming, and M. Valenzuela, "Cognitive Training for Post-Acute Traumatic Brain Injury: A Systematic Review and Meta-Analysis," *Frontiers in Human Neuroscience*, Vol. 10, October 2016, article 537.

Hart, B. B., L. K. Weaver, A. Gupta, S. H. Wilson, A. Vijayarangan, K. Deru, and D. Hebert, "Hyperbaric Oxygen for mTBI-Associated PCS and PTSD: Pooled Analysis of Results from Department of Defense and Other Published Studies," *Undersea and Hyperbaric Medicine*, Vol. 46, No. 3, February 2019, pp. 353–383.

Hassett, L., A. M. Moseley, and A. R. Harmer, "Fitness Training for Cardiorespiratory Conditioning After Traumatic Brain Injury," *Cochrane Database of Systematic Reviews*, Vol. 12, No. 12, December 29, 2017, article CD006123.

Health Resources and Services Administration, "Telehealth Licensing Requirements and Interstate Compacts," webpage, September 8, 2021. As of September 28, 2021: https://telehealth.hhs.gov/providers/policy-changes-during-the-covid-19-public-health-emergency/telehealth-licensing-requirements-and-interstate-compacts/

Hellewell, S. C., C. S. Beaton, T. Welton, and S. M. Grieve, "Characterizing the Risk of Depression Following Mild Traumatic Brain Injury: A Meta-Analysis of the Literature Comparing Chronic mTBI to Non-mTBI Populations," *Frontiers in Neurology*, Vol. 11, 2020, article 350.

Hellweg, S., and S. Johannes, "Physiotherapy After Traumatic Brain Injury: A Systematic Review of the Literature," *Brain Injury*, Vol. 22, No. 5, May 2008, pp. 365–373.

Hesdorffer, Dale C., Scott L. Rauch, and Carol A. Tamminga, "Long-Term Psychiatric Outcomes Following Traumatic Brain Injury: A Review of the Literature," *Journal of Head Trauma Rehabilitation*, Vol. 24, No. 6, November–December 2009, pp. 452–459.

Hicks, A. J., F. J. Clay, M. Hopwood, A. C. James, M. Jayaram, R. Batty, L. A. Perry, and J. L. Ponsford, "Efficacy and Harms of Pharmacological Interventions for Neurobehavioral Symptoms in Post-Traumatic Amnesia After Traumatic Brain Injury: A Systematic Review," *Journal of Neurotrauma*, Vol. 35, No. 23, December 2018, pp. 2755–2775.

Hicks, A. J., F. J. Clay, M. Hopwood, A. C. James, M. Jayaram, L. A. Perry, R. Batty, and J. L. Ponsford, "The Efficacy and Harms of Pharmacological Interventions for Aggression After Traumatic Brain Injury-Systematic Review," *Frontiers in Neurology*, Vol. 10, 2019, article 1169.

Hicks, A. J., F. J. Clay, M. Hopwood, A. C. James, L. A. Perry, M. Jayaram, R. Batty, and J. L. Ponsford, "Efficacy and Harms of Pharmacological Interventions for Anxiety After Traumatic Brain Injury: Systematic Review," *Journal of Neurotrauma*, Vol. 38, No. 5, March 2021, pp. 519–528.

Hicks, A. J., F. J. Clay, J. L. Ponsford, L. A. Perry, M. Jayaram, R. Batty, and M. Hopwood, "Pharmacotherapy for the Pseudobulbar Affect in Individuals Who Have Sustained a Traumatic Brain Injury: A Systematic Review," *Neuropsychology Review*, Vol. 30, No. 1, March 2020, pp. 28–50.

Hoge, C. W., D. McGurk, J. L. Thomas, A. L. Cox, C. C. Engel, and C. A. Castro, "Mild Traumatic Brain Injury in U.S. Soldiers Returning from Iraq," *New England Journal of Medicine*, Vol. 358, No. 5, 2008, pp. 453–463.

Huang, C. H., C. W. Lin, Y. C. Lee, C. Y. Huang, R. Y. Huang, Y. C. Tai, K. W. Wang, S. N. Yang, Y. T. Sun, and H. K. Wang, "Is Traumatic Brain Injury a Risk Factor for Neurodegeneration? A Meta-Analysis of Population-Based Studies," *BMC Neurology*, Vol. 18, No. 1, November 5, 2018, article 184.

Hutchison, M. G., A. P. Di Battista, J. McCoskey, and S. E. Watling, "Systematic Review of Mental Health Measures Associated with Concussive and Subconcussive Head Trauma in Former Athletes," *International Journal of Psychophysiology*, Vol. 132, Part A, October 2018, pp. 55–61.

Iaccarino, Mary Alexis, Lisa Liang Philpotts, Ross Zafonte, and Joseph Biederman, "Stimulant Use in the Management of Mild Traumatic Brain Injury: A Qualitative Literature Review," *Journal of Attention Disorders*, Vol. 24, No. 2, 2020, pp. 309–317.

Iljazi, A., H. Ashina, H. M. Al-Khazali, R. B. Lipton, M. Ashina, H. W. Schytz, and S. Ashina, "Post-Traumatic Stress Disorder After Traumatic Brain Injury: A Systematic Review and Meta-Analysis," *Neurological Sciences*, Vol. 41, No. 10, October 2020, pp. 2737–2746.

Iruthayarajah, J., F. Alibrahim, S. Mehta, S. Janzen, A. McIntyre, and R. Teasell, "Cognitive Behavioural Therapy for Aggression Among Individuals with Moderate to Severe Acquired Brain Injury: A Systematic Review and Meta-Analysis," *Brain Injury*, Vol. 32, No. 12, 2018, pp. 1443–1449.

Jafari, S., M. Etminan, F. Aminzadeh, and A. Samii, "Head Injury and Risk of Parkinson Disease: A Systematic Review and Meta-Analysis," *Movement Disorders*, Vol. 28, No. 9, August 2013, pp. 1222–1229.

Jin, C., and R. Schachar, "Methylphenidate Treatment of Attention-Deficit/Hyperactivity Disorder Secondary to Traumatic Brain Injury: A Critical Appraisal of Treatment Studies," *CNS Spectrums*, Vol. 9, No. 3, March 2004, pp. 217–226.

Julien, J., S. Joubert, M. C. Ferland, L. C. Frenette, M. M. Boudreau-Duhaime, L. Malo-Véronneau, and E. de Guise, "Association of Traumatic Brain Injury and Alzheimer Disease Onset: A Systematic Review," *Annals of Physical Rehabilitation Medicine*, Vol. 60, No. 5, September 2017, pp. 347–356.

Kennedy, M. R. T., C. Coelho, L. Turkstra, M. Ylvisaker, M. Moore Sohlberg, K. Yorkston, H. H. Chiou, and P. F. Kan, "Intervention for Executive Functions After Traumatic Brain Injury: A Systematic Review, Meta-Analysis and Clinical Recommendations," *Neuropsychological Rehabilitation*, Vol. 18, No. 3, June 2008, pp. 257–299.

Kim, H., and A. Colantonio, "Effectiveness of Rehabilitation in Enhancing Community Integration After Acute Traumatic Brain Injury: A Systematic Review," *American Journal of Occupational Therapy*, Vol. 64, No. 5, September–October 2010, pp. 709–719.

Kim, J. J., and A. D. Gean, "Imaging for the Diagnosis and Management of Traumatic Brain Injury," *Neurotherapeutics*, Vol. 8, No. 1, January 2011, pp. 39–53.

Kinne, B. L., J. L. Bott, N. M. Cron, and R. L. Iaquaniello, "Effectiveness of Vestibular Rehabilitation on Concussion-Induced Vertigo: A Systematic Review," *Physical Therapy Reviews*, Vol. 23, No. 6, November 2018, pp. 338–347.

Kohnen, R. F., D. L. Gerritsen, O. M. Smals, J. C. M. Lavrijsen, and Raymond T. C. M. Koopmans, "Prevalence of Neuropsychiatric Symptoms and Psychotropic Drug Use in Patients with Acquired Brain Injury in Long-Term Care: A Systematic Review," *Brain Injury*, Vol. 32, No. 13–14, 2018, pp. 1591–1600.

Kreitzer, N., R. Ancona, C. McCullumsmith, B. G. Kurowski, B. Foreman, L. B. Ngwenya, and O. Adeoye, "The Effect of Antidepressants on Depression After Traumatic Brain Injury: A Meta-Analysis," *Journal of Head Trauma Rehabilitation*, Vol. 34, No. 3, May–June 2019, pp. E47–E54.

Kroenke, K., R. L. Spitzer, and J. B. Williams, "The PHQ-9: Validity of a Brief Depression Severity Measure," *Journal of General Internal Medicine*, Vol. 16, No. 9, September 2001, pp. 606–613.

Kumar, K. S., S. Samuelkamaleshkumar, A. Viswanathan, and A. S. Macaden, "Cognitive Rehabilitation for Adults with Traumatic Brain Injury to Improve Occupational Outcomes," *Cochrane Database of Systematic Reviews*, Vol. 6, No. 6, June 20, 2017, article CD007935.

Lambez, B., and E. Vakil, "The Effectiveness of Memory Remediation Strategies After Traumatic Brain Injury: Systematic Review and Meta-Analysis," *Annals of Physical and Rehabilitation Medicine*, Vol. 64, No. 5, September 2021, article 101530.

Lane-Brown, A., and R. Tate, "Interventions for Apathy After Traumatic Brain Injury," *Cochrane Database of Systematic Reviews*, Vol. 2009, No. 2, April 15, 2009a, article CD006341.

———, "Apathy After Acquired Brain Impairment: A Systematic Review of Non-Pharmacological Interventions," *Neuropsychological Rehabilitation*, Vol. 19, No. 4, August 2009b, pp. 481–516.

Lannin, N. A., K. Laver, K. Henry, M. Turnbull, M. Elder, J. Campisi, J. Schmidt, and E. Schneider, "Effects of Case Management After Brain Injury: A Systematic Review," *NeuroRehabilitation*, Vol. 35, No. 4, 2014, pp. 635–641.

Lannin, Natasha A., and Annie McCluskey, "A Systematic Review of Upper Limb Rehabilitation for Adults with Traumatic Brain Injury," *Brain Impairment*, Vol. 9, No. 3, 2008, pp. 237–246.

Lauzier, F., A. F. Turgeon, A. Boutin, M. Shemilt, I. Côté, O. Lachance, P. M. Archambault, F. Lamontagne, L. Moore, F. Bernard, C. Gagnon, and D. Cook, "Clinical Outcomes, Predictors, and Prevalence of Anterior Pituitary Disorders Following Traumatic Brain Injury: A Systematic Review," *Critical Care Medicine*, Vol. 42, No. 3, March 2014, pp. 712–721.

Lee, Katherine M., Trisha L. Khatri, and Elizabeth R. Fudge, "US Department of Defense Warfighter Brain Health Initiative: Maximizing Performance on and off the Battlefield," *Journal of the American Association of Nurse Practitioners*, Vol. 32, No. 11, November 2020, pp. 720–728.

Leopold, A., A. Lourie, H. Petras, and E. Elias, "The Use of Assistive Technology for Cognition to Support the Performance of Daily Activities for Individuals with Cognitive Disabilities Due to Traumatic Brain Injury: The Current State of the Research," *NeuroRehabilitation*, Vol. 37, No. 3, 2015, pp. 359–378.

Lew, H. L., P. H. Lin, J. L. Fuh, S. J. Wang, D. J. Clark, and W. C. Walker, "Characteristics and Treatment of Headache After Traumatic Brain Injury: A Focused Review," *American Journal of Physical Medicine and Rehabilitation*, Vol. 85, No. 7, July 2006, pp. 619–627.

Li, Y., Y. Li, X. Li, S. Zhang, J. Zhao, X. Zhu, and G. Tian, "Head Injury as a Risk Factor for Dementia and Alzheimer's Disease: A Systematic Review and Meta-Analysis of 32 Observational Studies," *PLoS One*, Vol. 12, No. 1, 2017, article e0169650.

Lindquist, Lisa K., Holly C. Love, and Eric B. Elbogen, "Traumatic Brain Injury in Iraq and Afghanistan Veterans: New Results from a National Random Sample Study," *Journal of Neuropsychiatry and Clinical Neurosciences*, Vol. 29, No. 3, Summer 2017, pp. 254–259.

Little, A., C. Byrne, and R. Coetzer, "The Effectiveness of Cognitive Behaviour Therapy for Reducing Anxiety Symptoms Following Traumatic Brain Injury: A Meta-Analysis and Systematic Review," *NeuroRehabilitation*, Vol. 48, No. 1, 2021, pp. 67–82.

Liu, G., S. Ou, H. Cui, X. Li, Z. Yin, D. Gu, and Z. Wang, "Head Injury and Amyotrophic Lateral Sclerosis: A Meta-Analysis," *Neuroepidemiology*, Vol. 55, February 23, 2021, pp. 11–19.

Liu, Z. Q., X. Zeng, and C. Y. Duan, "Neuropsychological Rehabilitation and Psychotherapy of Adult Traumatic Brain Injury Patients with Depression: A Systematic Review and Meta-Analysis," *Journal of Neurosurgical Science*, Vol. 62, No. 1, February 2018, pp. 24–35.

LoBue, C., C. M. Cullum, N. Didehbani, K. Yeatman, B. Jones, M. A. Kraut, and J. Hart, Jr., "Neurodegenerative Dementias After Traumatic Brain Injury," *Journal of Neuropsychiatry and Clinical Neurosciences*, Vol. 30, No. 1, Winter 2018, pp. 7–13.

Loignon, A., M. C. Ouellet, and G. Belleville, "A Systematic Review and Meta-Analysis on PTSD Following TBI Among Military/Veteran and Civilian Populations," *Journal of Head Trauma Rehabilitation*, Vol. 35, No. 1, January–February 2020, pp. E21–E35.

Long-Term Impact of Military-Relevant Brain Injury Consortium – Chronic Effects of Neurotrauma Consortium, "About," webpage, undated. As of November 29, 2021: https://www.limbic-cenc.org/index.php/about/

Lowe, A., M. Bailey, T. O'Shaughnessy, and V. Macavei, "Treatment of Sleep Disturbance Following Stroke and Traumatic Brain Injury: A Systematic Review of Conservative Interventions," *Disability and Rehabilitation*, December 11, 2020, pp. 1–13.

Lyons, M. W. H., and W. J. Blackshaw, "Does Magnesium Sulfate Have a Role in the Management of Severe Traumatic Brain Injury in Civilian and Military Populations? A Systematic Review and Meta-Analysis," *Journal of the Royal Army Medical Corps*, Vol. 164, No. 6, November 2018, pp. 442–449.

Mahan, Steven, Rebecca Rous, and Anna Adlam, "Systematic Review of Neuropsychological Rehabilitation for Prospective Memory Deficits as a Consequence of Acquired Brain Injury," *Journal of the International Neuropsychological Society*, Vol. 23, No. 3, March 2017, pp. 254–265.

Makdissi, M., K. J. Schneider, N. Feddermann-Demont, K. M. Guskiewicz, S. Hinds, J. J. Leddy, M. McCrea, M. Turner, and K. M. Johnston, "Approach to Investigation and Treatment of Persistent Symptoms Following Sport-Related Concussion: A Systematic Review," *British Journal of Sports Medicine*, Vol. 51, No. 12, June 2017, pp. 958–968.

Maksimowski, M. B., and R. R. Tampi, "Efficacy of Stimulants for Psychiatric Symptoms in Individuals with Traumatic Brain Injury," *Annals of Clinical Psychiatry*, Vol. 28, No. 3, August 2016, pp. 156–166.

Manivannan, S., M. Al-Amri, M. Postans, L. J. Westacott, W. Gray, and M. Zaben, "The Effectiveness of Virtual Reality Interventions for Improvement of Neurocognitive Performance After Traumatic Brain Injury: A Systematic Review," *Journal of Head Trauma Rehabilitation*, Vol. 34, No. 2, March–April 2019, pp. E52–E65.

Manley, G., A. J. Gardner, K. J. Schneider, K. M. Guskiewicz, J. Bailes, R. C. Cantu, R. J. Castellani, M. Turner, B. D. Jordan, C. Randolph, J. Dvořák, K. A. Hayden, C. H. Tator, P. McCrory, and G. L. Iverson, "A Systematic Review of Potential Long-Term Effects of Sport-Related Concussion," *British Journal of Sports Medicine*, Vol. 51, No. 12, June 2017, pp. 969–977.

Marras, C., C. A. Hincapié, V. L. Kristman, C. Cancelliere, S. Soklaridis, A. Li, J. Borg, J. L. af Geijerstam, and J. D. Cassidy, "Systematic Review of the Risk of Parkinson's Disease After Mild Traumatic Brain Injury: Results of the International Collaboration on Mild Traumatic Brain Injury Prognosis," *Archives of Physical Medicine and Rehabilitation*, Vol. 95, No. 3 Supp., March 2014, pp. S238–S244.

Marshall, Shawn, Robert Teasell, Nestor Bayona, Corbin Lippert, Josie Chundamala, James Villamere, David Mackie, Nora Cullen, and Mark Bayley, "Motor Impairment Rehabilitation Post Acquired Brain Injury," *Brain Injury*, Vol. 21, No. 2, February 2007, pp. 133–160.

Mast, H., A. Mendelson, M. Möddel, and J. Kejda-Scharler, "Association traumatismes crâniocérébraux légers avec troubles cognitifs chroniques et lésions encéphaliques axonales diffuses" ["Association of Mild Traumatic Brain Injury with Chronic Cognitive Changes and Diffuse Axonal Injury"], *Douleur et Analgésie*, Vol. 26, No. Supp. 1, 2013, pp. S28–S31.

Matarazzo, Bridget B., Hal S. Wortzel, Brooke A. Dorsey Holliman, and Lisa A. Brenner, "Evidence-Based Intervention Strategies for Veterans and Military Personnel with Traumatic Brain Injury and Co-Morbid Mental Health Conditions: A Systematic Review," *Brain Impairment*, Vol. 14, No. 1, 2013, pp. 42–50.

McAllister, Thomas W., "Neurobiological Consequences of Traumatic Brain Injury," *Dialogues in Clinical Neuroscience*, Vol. 13, No. 3, 2011, pp. 287–300.

McCabe, Pat, Corbin Lippert, Margaret Weiser, Maureen Hilditch, Cheryl Hartridge, and James Villamere, "Community Reintegration Following Acquired Brain Injury," *Brain Injury*, Vol. 21, No. 2, February 2007, pp. 231–257.

McCrea, M., G. L. Iverson, T. W. McAllister, T. A. Hammeke, M. R. Powell, W. B. Barr, and J. P. Kelly, "An Integrated Review of Recovery After Mild Traumatic Brain Injury (MTBI): Implications for Clinical Management," *Clinical Neuropsychologist*, Vol. 23, No. 8, November 2009, pp. 1368–1390.

McDonnell, M. N., A. E. Smith, and S. F. Mackintosh, "Aerobic Exercise to Improve Cognitive Function in Adults with Neurological Disorders: A Systematic Review," *Archives of Physical Medicine and Rehabilitation*, Vol. 92, No. 7, July 2011, pp. 1044–1052.

McPherson, A. L., T. Nagai, K. E. Webster, and T. E. Hewett, "Musculoskeletal Injury Risk After Sport-Related Concussion: A Systematic Review and Meta-Analysis," *American Journal of Sports Medicine*, Vol. 47, No. 7, June 2019, pp. 1754–1762.

Merezhinskaya, N., R. K. Mallia, D. Park, D. W. Bryden, K. Mathur, and F. M. Barker II, "Visual Deficits and Dysfunctions Associated with Traumatic Brain Injury: A Systematic Review and Meta-Analysis," *Optometry and Vision Science*, Vol. 96, No. 8, August 2019, pp. 542–555.

Merritt, V. C., S. M. Jurick, L. D. Crocker, M. J. Sullan, M. S. Sakamoto, D. K. Davey, S. N. Hoffman, A. V. Keller, and A. J. Jak, "Associations Between Multiple Remote Mild TBIs and Objective Neuropsychological Functioning and Subjective Symptoms in Combat-Exposed Veterans," *Archives of Clinical Neuropsychology*, Vol. 35, No. 5, August 2020, pp. 491–505.

Meshkini, A., M. Meshkini, and H. Sadeghi-Bazargani, "Citicoline for Traumatic Brain Injury: A Systematic Review & Meta-Analysis," *Journal of Injury and Violence Research*, Vol. 9, No. 1, January 2017, pp. 41–50.

Mikolić, A., S. Polinder, I. R. A. Retel Helmrich, J. A. Haagsma, and M. C. Cnossen, "Treatment for Posttraumatic Stress Disorder in Patients with a History of Traumatic Brain Injury: A Systematic Review," *Clinical Psychology Review*, Vol. 73, November 2019, article 101776.

Military Health System, "DOD TBI Worldwide Numbers," webpage, undated-a. As of August 30, 2021:
https://health.mil/About-MHS/OASDHA/Defense-Health-Agency/Research-and-Development/Traumatic-Brain-Injury-Center-of-Excellence/DOD-TBI-Worldwide-Numbers

———, "Publications," webpage, undated-b. As of August 30, 2021:
https://health.mil/Reference-Center/Publications?refVector=000000000001000&refSrc=139

Minen, M., S. Jinich, and G. Vallespir Ellett, "Behavioral Therapies and Mind-Body Interventions for Posttraumatic Headache and Post-Concussive Symptoms: A Systematic Review," *Headache*, Vol. 59, No. 2, February 2019, pp. 151–163.

Mohamed, Mona Salah, Iman El Sayed, Adel Zaki, and Sherif Abdelmonem, "Assessment of the Effect of Amantadine in Patients with Traumatic Brain Injury: A Meta-Analysis," *Journal of Trauma and Acute Care Surgery*, July 20, 2021.

Mollayeva, T., T. Kendzerska, S. Mollayeva, C. M. Shapiro, A. Colantonio, and J. D. Cassidy, "A Systematic Review of Fatigue in Patients with Traumatic Brain Injury: The Course, Predictors and Consequences," *Neuroscience and Biobehavioral Reviews*, Vol. 47, November 2014, pp. 684–716.

Möller, M. C., J. Lexell, and K. Wilbe Ramsay, "Effectiveness of Specialized Rehabilitation After Mild Traumatic Brain Injury: A Systematic Review and Meta-Analysis," *Journal of Rehabilitation Medicine*, Vol. 53, No. 2, February 5, 2021, article jrm00149.

Mollica, A., F. Safavifar, M. Fralick, P. Giacobbe, N. Lipsman, and M. J. Burke, "Transcranial Magnetic Stimulation for the Treatment of Concussion: A Systematic Review," *Neuromodulation*, Vol. 24, No. 5, July 2021, pp. 803–812.

Molloy, C., R. M. Conroy, D. R. Cotter, and M. Cannon, "Is Traumatic Brain Injury a Risk Factor for Schizophrenia? A Meta-Analysis of Case-Controlled Population-Based Studies," *Schizophrenia Bulletin*, Vol. 37, No. 6, November 2011, pp. 1104–1110.

Morris, R. P., J. C. Fletcher-Smith, and K. A. Radford, "A Systematic Review of Peer Mentoring Interventions for People with Traumatic Brain Injury," *Clinical Rehabilitation*, Vol. 31, No. 8, August 2017, pp. 1030–1038.

Morris, T., J. G. Osman, J. M. T. Muñoz, D. C. Miserachs, and A. P. Leone, "The Role of Physical Exercise in Cognitive Recovery After Traumatic Brain Injury: A Systematic Review," *Restorative Neurology and Neuroscience*, Vol. 34, No. 6, November 2016, pp. 977–988.

Mueller, C., S. Wesenberg, F. Nestmann, B. Stubbs, P. Bebbington, and V. Raymont, "Interventions to Enhance Coping After Traumatic Brain Injury: A Systematic Review," *International Journal of Therapy and Rehabilitation*, Vol. 25, No. 3, March 2018, pp. 107–119.

Murray, D. A., D. Meldrum, and O. Lennon, "Can Vestibular Rehabilitation Exercises Help Patients with Concussion? A Systematic Review of Efficacy, Prescription and Progression Patterns," *British Journal of Sports Medicine*, Vol. 51, No. 5, March 2017, pp. 442–451.

Nampiaparampil, D. E., "Prevalence of Chronic Pain After Traumatic Brain Injury: A Systematic Review," *JAMA*, Vol. 300, No. 6, August 2008, pp. 711–719.

Narapareddy, B. R., L. Narapareddy, A. Lin, S. Wigh, J. Nanavati, J. Dougherty III, M. Nowrangi, and D. Roy, "Treatment of Depression After Traumatic Brain Injury: A Systematic Review Focused on Pharmacological and Neuromodulatory Interventions," *Psychosomatics*, Vol. 61, No. 5, September–October 2020, pp. 481–497.

National Center for Veterans Analysis and Statistics, "Profile of Post-9/11 Veterans: 2016," briefing slides, March 2018.

National Collegiate Athletic Association, "NCAA-DOD CARE Consortium," webpage, undated. As of November 29, 2021:
https://www.ncaa.org/sport-science-institute/topics/ncaa-dod-care-consortium

National Institute of Child Health and Human Development, "Traumatic Brain Injury (TBI) Resources," webpage, undated. As of November 1, 2021:
https://www.nichd.nih.gov/health/topics/tbi/more_information/resources

National Institute of Mental Health, "Panic Disorder," webpage, undated-a. As of August 30, 2021:
https://www.nimh.nih.gov/health/statistics/panic-disorder

———, "Schizophrenia," webpage, undated-b. As of August 30, 2021:
https://www.nimh.nih.gov/health/statistics/schizophrenia

Novack, T. A., A. L. Alderson, B. A. Bush, J. M. Meythaler, and K. Canupp, "Cognitive and Functional Recovery at 6 and 12 Months Post-TBI," *Brain Injury*, Vol. 14, No. 11, November 2000, pp. 987–996.

Novack, T. A., B. A. Bush, J. M. Meythaler, and K. Canupp, "Outcome After Traumatic Brain Injury: Pathway Analysis of Contributions from Premorbid, Injury Severity, and Recovery Variables," *Archives of Physical Medicine and Rehabilitation*, Vol. 82, No. 3, March 2001, pp. 300–305.

Nygren-de Boussard, C., L. W. Holm, C. Cancelliere, A. K. Godbolt, E. Boyle, B. M. Stålnacke, C. A. Hincapié, J. D. Cassidy, and J. Borg, "Nonsurgical Interventions After Mild Traumatic Brain Injury: A Systematic Review. Results of the International Collaboration on Mild Traumatic Brain Injury Prognosis," *Archives of Physical Medicine and Rehabilitation*, Vol. 95, No. 3, Supp., March 2014, pp. S257–S264.

O'Carroll, G. C., S. L. King, S. Carroll, J. L. Perry, and N. Vanicek, "The Effects of Exercise to Promote Quality of Life in Individuals with Traumatic Brain Injuries: A Systematic Review," *Brain Injury*, Vol. 34, No. 13–14, December 2020, pp. 1701–1713.

Office of Data Governance and Analytics, *Minority Veterans Report: Military Service History and VA Benefit Utilization Statistics*, Washington, D.C.: U.S. Department of Veterans Affairs, March 2017.

O'Neil, M. E., K. F. Carlson, H. K. Holmer, C. K. Ayers, B. J. Morasco, D. Kansagara, and K. Kondo, *Chronic Pain in Veterans and Servicemembers with a History of Mild Traumatic Brain Injury: A Systematic Review*, Washington, D.C.: U.S. Department of Veterans Affairs, 2020.

O'Neil, M. E., K. Carlson, D. Storzbach, L. Brenner, M. Freeman, A. Quiñones, M. Motu'apuaka, M. Ensley, and D. Kansagara, *Complications of Mild Traumatic Brain Injury in Veterans and Military Personnel: A Systematic Review*, Washington, D.C.: U.S. Department of Veterans Affairs, 2013.

O'Neil, Maya E., Kathleen F. Carlson, Daniel Storzbach, Lisa A. Brenner, Michele Freeman, Ana R. Quiñones, Makalapua Motu'apuaka, and Devan Kansagara, "Factors Associated with Mild Traumatic Brain Injury in Veterans and Military Personnel: A Systematic Review," *Journal of the International Neuropsychological Society*, Vol. 20, No. 3, March 2014, pp. 249–261.

O'Neil-Pirozzi, T. M., M. R. Kennedy, and M. M. Sohlberg, "Evidence-Based Practice for the Use of Internal Strategies as a Memory Compensation Technique After Brain Injury: A Systematic Review," *Journal of Head Trauma Rehabilitation*, Vol. 31, No. 4, July–August 2016, pp. E1–E11.

O'Sullivan, Michelle, Emily Glorney, Annette Sterr, Michael Oddy, and Sara da Silva Ramos, "Traumatic Brain Injury and Violent Behavior in Females: A Systematic Review," *Aggression and Violent Behavior*, Vol. 25, Part A, November–December 2015, pp. 54–64.

Ownsworth, T., U. Arnautovska, E. Beadle, D. H. K. Shum, and W. Moyle, "Efficacy of Telerehabilitation for Adults with Traumatic Brain Injury: A Systematic Review," *Journal of Head Trauma Rehabilitation*, Vol. 33, No. 4, July–August 2018, pp. E33–E46.

Ownsworth, T., and C. Haslam, "Impact of Rehabilitation on Self-Concept Following Traumatic Brain Injury: An Exploratory Systematic Review of Intervention Methodology and Efficacy," *Neuropsychological Rehabilitation*, Vol. 26, No. 1, 2016, pp. 1–35.

Oyesanya, Tolu O., and Earlise C. Ward, "Mental Health in Women with Traumatic Brain Injury: A Systematic Review on Depression and Hope," *Health Care for Women International*, Vol. 37, No. 1, 2016, pp. 45–74.

Ozolins, B., N. Aimers, L. Parrington, and A. J. Pearce, "Movement Disorders and Motor Impairments Following Repeated Head Trauma: A Systematic Review of the Literature 1990–2015," *Brain Injury*, Vol. 30, No. 8, 2016, pp. 937–947.

Paice, L., A. Aleligay, and M. Checklin, "A Systematic Review of Interventions for Adults with Social Communication Impairments Due to an Acquired Brain Injury: Significant Other Reports," *International Journal of Speech-Language Pathology*, Vol. 22, No. 5, October 2020, pp. 537–548.

Paraschakis, A., and A. H. Katsanos, "Antidepressants for Depression Associated with Traumatic Brain Injury: A Meta-Analytical Study of Randomised Controlled Trials," *East Asian Archives of Psychiatry*, Vol. 27, No. 4, December 2017, pp. 142–149.

Park, H. Y., K. Maitra, and K. M. Martinez, "The Effect of Occupation-Based Cognitive Rehabilitation for Traumatic Brain Injury: A Meta-Analysis of Randomized Controlled Trials," *Occupational Therapy International*, Vol. 22, No. 2, June 2015, pp. 104–116.

Parker, K., A. Cilluffo, and R. Stepler, "6 Facts About the U.S. Military and Its Changing Demographics," Pew Research Center, April 13, 2017.

Pattinson, C. L., and J. M. Gill, "Risk of Dementia After TBI—A Cause of Growing Concern," *Nature Reviews Neurology*, Vol. 14, No. 9, September 2018, pp. 511–512.

Peppel, L. D., G. M. Ribbers, and M. H. Heijenbrok-Kal, "Pharmacological and Non-Pharmacological Interventions for Depression After Moderate-to-Severe Traumatic Brain Injury: A Systematic Review and Meta-Analysis," *Journal of Neurotrauma*, Vol. 37, No. 14, July 2020, pp. 1587–1596.

Perl, Daniel P., "Military TBI: Is It the Same as Civilian TBI?" *The Bridge*, Vol. 46, No. 1, Spring 2016, pp. 65–68.

Perry, D. C., V. E. Sturm, M. J. Peterson, C. F. Pieper, T. Bullock, B. F. Boeve, B. L. Miller, K. M. Guskiewicz, M. S. Berger, J. H. Kramer, and K. A. Welsh-Bohmer, "Association of Traumatic Brain Injury with Subsequent Neurological and Psychiatric Disease: A Meta-Analysis," *Journal of Neurosurgery*, Vol. 124, No. 2, February 2016, pp. 511–526.

Perry, S. A., R. Coetzer, and C. W. N. Saville, "The Effectiveness of Physical Exercise as an Intervention to Reduce Depressive Symptoms Following Traumatic Brain Injury: A Meta-Analysis and Systematic Review," *Neuropsychological Rehabilitation*, Vol. 30, No. 3, April 2020, pp. 564–578.

Peterson, K., S. Veazie, D. Bourne, and J. Anderson, "Association Between Traumatic Brain Injury and Dementia in Veterans: A Rapid Systematic Review," *Journal of Head Trauma Rehabilitation*, Vol. 35, No. 3, May–June 2020, pp. 198–208.

Pilon, L., N. Frankenmolen, and D. Bertens, "Treatments for Sleep Disturbances in Individuals with Acquired Brain Injury: A Systematic Review," *Clinical Rehabilitation*, Vol. 35, No. 11, November 2021, pp. 1518–1529.

Pinto, Joana O., Artemisa R. Dores, Bruno Peixoto, Andreia Geraldo, and Fernando Barbosa, "Systematic Review of Sensory Stimulation Programs in the Rehabilitation of Acquired Brain Injury," *European Psychologist*, November 30, 2020.

Polinder, S., J. A. Haagsma, D. van Klaveren, E. W. Steyerberg, and E. F. van Beeck, "Health-Related Quality of Life After TBI: A Systematic Review of Study Design, Instruments, Measurement Properties, and Outcome," *Population Health Metrics*, Vol. 13, February 2015, article 4.

Postol, N., J. Marquez, S. Spartalis, A. Bivard, and N. J. Spratt, "Do Powered Over-Ground Lower Limb Robotic Exoskeletons Affect Outcomes in the Rehabilitation of People with Acquired Brain Injury?" *Disability and Rehabilitation, Assistive Technology*, Vol. 14, No. 8, November 2019, pp. 764–775.

Powell, J. M., T. J. Rich, and E. K. Wise, "Effectiveness of Occupation- and Activity-Based Interventions to Improve Everyday Activities and Social Participation for People with Traumatic Brain Injury: A Systematic Review," *American Journal of Occupational Therapy*, Vol. 70, No. 3, May–June 2016.

Pugh, Mary Jo, Erin P. Finley, Chen-Pin Wang, Laurel A. Copeland, Carlos A. Jaramillo, Alicia A. Swan, Christine A. Elnitsky, Luci K. Leykum, Eric M. Mortensen, and Blessen A. Eapen, "A Retrospective Cohort Study of Comorbidity Trajectories Associated with Traumatic Brain Injury in Veterans of the Iraq and Afghanistan Wars," *Brain Injury*, Vol. 30, No. 12, 2016, pp. 1481–1490.

Radomski, M. V., M. Anheluk, M. P. Bartzen, and J. Zola, "Effectiveness of Interventions to Address Cognitive Impairments and Improve Occupational Performance After Traumatic Brain Injury: A Systematic Review," *American Journal of Occupational Therapy*, Vol. 70, No. 3, May–June 2016.

Rahmani, E., T. M. Lemelle, E. Samarbafzadeh, and A. S. Kablinger, "Pharmacological Treatment of Agitation and/or Aggression in Patients with Traumatic Brain Injury: A Systematic Review of Reviews," *Journal of Head Trauma Rehabilitation*, Vol. 36, No. 4, July–August 2021, pp. E262–E283.

Renzenbrink, G. J., J. H. Buurke, A. V. Nene, A. C. Geurts, G. Kwakkel, and J. S. Rietman, "Improving Walking Capacity by Surgical Correction of Equinovarus Foot Deformity in Adult Patients with Stroke or Traumatic Brain Injury: A Systematic Review," *Journal of Rehabilitation Medicine*, Vol. 44, No. 8, July 2012, pp. 614–623.

Reyes, N. G. D., A. I. Espiritu, and V. M. M. Anlacan, "Efficacy of Sertraline in Post-Traumatic Brain Injury (Post-TBI) Depression and Quality of Life: A Systematic Review and Meta-Analysis of Randomized Controlled Trials," *Clinical Neurology and Neurosurgery*, Vol. 181, June 2019, pp. 104–111.

Rickardsson, Nils, Daniel Stopforth, and David Gillanders, "Remotely Delivered Interventions for Caregivers of Adults with Acquired Brain Injuries: A Systematic Review," submission record, PROSPERO, 2020. As of October 20, 2021:
https://www.crd.york.ac.uk/prospero/display_record.php?ID=CRD42020189235

Rietdijk, R., L. Togher, and E. Power, "Supporting Family Members of People with Traumatic Brain Injury Using Telehealth: A Systematic Review," *Journal of Rehabilitation Medicine*, Vol. 44, No. 11, November 2012, pp. 913–921.

Rodríguez-Rajo, P., D. Leno Colorado, A. Enseñat-Cantallops, and A. García-Molina, "Rehabilitation of Social Cognition Impairment After Traumatic Brain Injury: A Systematic Review," *Neurologia* (English ed.), December 12, 2018.

Rogers, Jeffrey M., and Christina A. Read, "Psychiatric Comorbidity Following Traumatic Brain Injury," *Brain Injury*, Vol. 21, No. 13–14, December 2007, pp. 1321–1333.

Rohling, M. L., M. E. Faust, B. Beverly, and G. Demakis, "Effectiveness of Cognitive Rehabilitation Following Acquired Brain Injury: A Meta-Analytic Re-Examination of Cicerone et al.'s (2000, 2005) Systematic Reviews," *Neuropsychology*, Vol. 23, No. 1, January 2009, pp. 20–39.

Roitsch, Jane, Rachael Redman, Anne M. P. Michalek, Rachel K. Johnson, and Anastasia M. Raymer, "Quality Appraisal of Systematic Reviews for Behavioral Treatments of Attention Disorders in Traumatic Brain Injury," *Journal of Head Trauma Rehabilitation*, Vol. 34, No. 4, July–August 2019, pp. E42–E50.

Ruff, R., "Two Decades of Advances in Understanding of Mild Traumatic Brain Injury," *Journal of Head Trauma Rehabilitation*, Vol. 20, No. 1, January–February 2005, pp. 5–18.

Rutherford, George W., and Renee C. Wlodarczyk, "Distant Sequelae of Traumatic Brain Injury: Premature Mortality and Intracranial Neoplasms," *Journal of Head Trauma Rehabilitation*, Vol. 24, No. 6, November–December 2009, pp. 468–474.

Ruttan, L., K. Martin, A. Liu, B. Colella, and R. E. Green, "Long-Term Cognitive Outcome in Moderate to Severe Traumatic Brain Injury: A Meta-Analysis Examining Timed and Untimed Tests at 1 and 4.5 or More Years After Injury," *Archives of Physical Medicine and Rehabilitation*, Vol. 89, No. 12, Supp., December 2008, pp. S69–S76.

Ryan, G. W., and H. R. Bernard, "Techniques to Identify Themes," *Field Methods*, Vol. 15, No. 1, 2003, pp. 85–109.

Salter, K. L., J. A. McClure, N. C. Foley, K. Sequeira, and R. W. Teasell, "Pharmacotherapy for Depression Posttraumatic Brain Injury: A Meta-Analysis," *Journal of Head Trauma Rehabilitation*, Vol. 31, No. 4, July–August 2016, pp. E21–E32.

Sami, M. B., and R. Faruqui, "The Effectiveness of Dopamine Agonists for Treatment of Neuropsychiatric Symptoms Post Brain Injury and Stroke," *Acta Neuropsychiatrica*, Vol. 27, No. 6, December 2015, pp. 317–326.

Šarkić, B., J. M. Douglas, and A. Simpson, "Peripheral Auditory Dysfunction Secondary to Traumatic Brain Injury: A Systematic Review of Literature," *Brain Injury*, Vol. 33, No. 2, January 2019, pp. 111–128.

Sawyer, Q., B. Vesci, and T. C. McLeod, "Physical Activity and Intermittent Postconcussion Symptoms After a Period of Symptom-Limited Physical and Cognitive Rest," *Journal of Athletic Training*, Vol. 51, No. 9, September 2016, pp. 739–742.

Schaffert, J., C. LoBue, L. Fields, K. Wilmoth, N. Didehbani, J. Hart, Jr., and C. M. Cullum, "Neuropsychological Functioning in Ageing Retired NFL Players: A Critical Review," *International Review of Psychiatry*, Vol. 32, No. 1, February 2020, pp. 71–88.

Schneider, H. J., I. Kreitschmann-Andermahr, E. Ghigo, G. K. Stalla, and A. Agha, "Hypothalamopituitary Dysfunction Following Traumatic Brain Injury and Aneurysmal Subarachnoid Hemorrhage: A Systematic Review," *JAMA*, Vol. 298, No. 12, September 2007, pp. 1429–1438.

Schneider, K. J., G. L. Iverson, C. A. Emery, P. McCrory, S. A. Herring, and W. H. Meeuwisse, "The Effects of Rest and Treatment Following Sport-Related Concussion: A Systematic Review of the Literature," *British Journal of Sports Medicine*, Vol. 47, No. 5, April 2013, pp. 304–307.

Scholten, A. C., J. A. Haagsma, M. C. Cnossen, M. Olff, E. F. van Beeck, and S. Polinder, "Prevalence of and Risk Factors for Anxiety and Depressive Disorders After Traumatic Brain Injury: A Systematic Review," *Journal of Neurotrauma*, Vol. 33, No. 22, November 2016, pp. 1969–1994.

Schretlen, D. J., and A. M. Shapiro, "A Quantitative Review of the Effects of Traumatic Brain Injury on Cognitive Functioning," *International Review of Psychiatry*, Vol. 15, No. 4, November 2003, pp. 341–349.

Schrijnemaekers, Anne-Claire, Sanne M. J. Smeets, Rudolf W. H. M. Ponds, Caroline M. van Heugten, and Sascha Rasquin, "Treatment of Unawareness of Deficits in Patients with Acquired Brain Injury: A Systematic Review," *Journal of Head Trauma Rehabilitation*, Vol. 29, No. 5, September–October 2014, pp. E9–E30.

Schultz, R., and R. L. Tate, "Methodological Issues in Longitudinal Research on Cognitive Recovery After Traumatic Brain Injury: Evidence from a Systematic Review," *Brain Impairment*, Vol. 14, No. 3, December 2013, pp. 450–474.

Sharma, B., D. Allison, P. Tucker, D. Mabbott, and B. W. Timmons, "Cognitive and Neural Effects of Exercise Following Traumatic Brain Injury: A Systematic Review of Randomized and Controlled Clinical Trials," *Brain Injury*, Vol. 34, No. 2, 2020, pp. 149–159.

Sheng, P., L. Hou, X. Wang, X. Wang, C. Huang, M. Yu, X. Han, and Y. Dong, "Efficacy of Modafinil on Fatigue and Excessive Daytime Sleepiness Associated with Neurological Disorders: A Systematic Review and Meta-Analysis," *PLoS One*, Vol. 8, No. 12, December 2013, article e81802.

Shepherd-Banigan, M. E., J. R. McDuffie, A. Shapiro, M. Brancu, N. Sperber, N. N. Mehta, C. H. Van Houtven, and J. W. Williams, Jr., *Interventions to Support Caregivers or Families of Patients with TBI, PTSD, or Polytrauma: A Systematic Review*, Washington, D.C.: U.S. Department of Veterans Affairs, February 2018.

Shepherd-Banigan, M. E., A. Shapiro, J. R. McDuffie, M. Brancu, N. R. Sperber, C. H. Van Houtven, A. S. Kosinski, N. N. Mehta, A. Nagi, and J. W. Williams, Jr., "Interventions That Support or Involve Caregivers or Families of Patients with Traumatic Injury: A Systematic Review," *Journal of General Internal Medicine*, Vol. 33, No. 7, July 2018, pp. 1177–1186.

Sigmundsdottir, Linda, Wendy A. Longley, and Robyn L. Tate, "Computerised Cognitive Training in Acquired Brain Injury: A Systematic Review of Outcomes Using the International Classification of Functioning (ICF)," *Neuropsychological Rehabilitation*, Vol. 26, No. 5–6, October 2016, pp. 673–741.

Simpson, Grahame, and Robyn Tate, "Suicidality in People Surviving a Traumatic Brain Injury: Prevalence, Risk Factors and Implications for Clinical Management," *Brain Injury*, Vol. 21, No. 13–14, December 2007, pp. 1335–1351.

Sivan, M., V. Neumann, R. Kent, A. Stroud, and B. B. Bhakta, "Pharmacotherapy for Treatment of Attention Deficits After Non-Progressive Acquired Brain Injury. A Systematic Review," *Clinical Rehabilitation*, Vol. 24, No. 2, February 2010, pp. 110–121.

Slowinski, A., R. Coetzer, and C. Byrne, "Pharmacotherapy Effectiveness in Treating Depression After Traumatic Brain Injury: A Meta-Analysis," *Journal of Neuropsychiatry and Clinical Neuroscience*, Vol. 31, No. 3, Summer 2019, pp. 220–227.

Snell, D. L., L. J. Surgenor, E. J. Hay-Smith, and R. J. Siegert, "A Systematic Review of Psychological Treatments for Mild Traumatic Brain Injury: An Update on the Evidence," *Journal of Clinical and Experimental Neuropsychology*, Vol. 31, No. 1, January 2009, pp. 20–38.

Snowden, T. M., A. K. Hinde, H. M. O. Reid, and B. R. Christie, "Does Mild Traumatic Brain Injury Increase the Risk for Dementia? A Systematic Review and Meta-Analysis," *Journal of Alzheimer's Disease*, Vol. 78, No. 2, 2020, pp. 757–775.

Soo, C., and R. Tate, "Psychological Treatment for Anxiety in People with Traumatic Brain Injury," *Cochrane Database of Systematic Reviews*, No. 3, July 18, 2007, article CD005239.

Spencer, L., R. Potterton, K. Allen, P. Musiat, and U. Schmidt, "Internet-Based Interventions for Carers of Individuals with Psychiatric Disorders, Neurological Disorders, or Brain Injuries: Systematic Review," *Journal of Medical Internet Research*, Vol. 21, No. 7, July 9, 2019, article e10876.

Spreij, Lauriane A., Johanna M. A. Visser-Meily, Caroline M. van Heugten, and Tanja C. W. Nijboer, "Novel Insights into the Rehabilitation of Memory Post Acquired Brain Injury: A Systematic Review," *Frontiers in Human Neuroscience*, Vol. 8, December 2014, article 993.

Srisurapanont, K., Y. Samakarn, B. Kamklong, P. Siratrairat, A. Bumiputra, M. Jaikwang, and M. Srisurapanont, "Blue-Wavelength Light Therapy for Post-Traumatic Brain Injury Sleepiness, Sleep Disturbance, Depression, and Fatigue: A Systematic Review and Network Meta-Analysis," *PLoS One*, Vol. 16, No. 2, February 2021, article e0246172.

Steel, Joanne, Elise Elbourn, and Leanne Togher, "Narrative Discourse Intervention After Traumatic Brain Injury: A Systematic Review of the Literature," *Topics in Language Disorders*, Vol. 41, No. 1, 2021, pp. 47–72.

Sullivan, K. A., H. Blaine, S. A. Kaye, A. Theadom, C. Haden, and S. S. Smith, "A Systematic Review of Psychological Interventions for Sleep and Fatigue After Mild Traumatic Brain Injury," *Journal of Neurotrauma*, Vol. 35, No. 2, January 2018, pp. 195–209.

Sullivan, K. A., S. A. Kaye, H. Blaine, S. L. Edmed, S. Meares, K. Rossa, and C. Haden, "Psychological Approaches for the Management of Persistent Postconcussion Symptoms After Mild Traumatic Brain Injury: A Systematic Review," *Disability and Rehabilitation*, Vol. 42, No. 16, August 2020, pp. 2243–2251.

Swedish Agency for Health Technology Assessment and Assessment of Social Services, *Rehabilitation for Adults with Traumatic Brain Injury: A Systematic Review and Assessment of Medical, Economic, Social and Ethical Aspects*, Stockholm, December 2019.

Synnot, A., M. Chau, V. Pitt, D. O'Connor, R. L. Gruen, J. Wasiak, O. Clavisi, L. Pattuwage, and K. Phillips, "Interventions for Managing Skeletal Muscle Spasticity Following Traumatic Brain Injury," *Cochrane Database of Systematic Reviews*, Vol. 11, No. 11, November 22, 2017, article CD008929.

Szarka, N., D. Szellar, S. Kiss, N. Farkas, Z. Szakacs, A. Czigler, Z. Ungvari, P. Hegyi, A. Buki, and P. Toth, "Effect of Growth Hormone on Neuropsychological Outcomes and Quality of Life of Patients with Traumatic Brain Injury: A Systematic Review," *Journal of Neurotrauma*, Vol. 38, No. 11, June 2021, pp. 1467–1483.

Tanielian, Terri, and Lisa H. Jaycox, eds., *Invisible Wounds of War: Psychological and Cognitive Injuries, Their Consequences, and Services to Assist Recovery*, Santa Monica, Calif.: RAND Corporation, MG-720-CCF, 2008. As of November 29, 2021: https://www.rand.org/pubs/monographs/MG720.html

Tarnutzer, A. A., D. Straumann, P. Brugger, and N. Feddermann-Demont, "Persistent Effects of Playing Football and Associated (Subconcussive) Head Trauma on Brain Structure and Function: A Systematic Review of the Literature," *British Journal of Sports Medicine*, Vol. 51, No. 22, November 2017, pp. 1592–1604.

Tate, Robyn, Donna Wakim, and Michelle Genders, "A Systematic Review of the Efficacy of Community-Based, Leisure/Social Activity Programmes for People with Traumatic Brain Injury," *Brain Impairment*, Vol. 15, No. 3, 2014, pp. 157–176.

Teo, S. H., K. N. K. Fong, Z. Chen, and R. C. K. Chung, "Cognitive and Psychological Interventions for the Reduction of Post-Concussion Symptoms in Patients with Mild Traumatic Brain Injury: A Systematic Review," *Brain Injury*, Vol. 34, No. 10, August 2020, pp. 1305–1321.

Terrio, H., L. A. Brenner, B. J. Ivins, J. M. Cho, K. Helmick, K. Schwab, K. Scally, R. Bretthauer, and D. Warden, "Traumatic Brain Injury Screening: Preliminary Findings in a US Army Brigade Combat Team," *Journal of Head Trauma Rehabilitation*, Vol. 24, No. 1, January–February 2009, pp. 14–23.

Thomas, R. E., J. Alves, M. M. Vaska Mlis, and R. Magalhaes, "Therapy and Rehabilitation of Mild Brain Injury/Concussion: Systematic Review," *Restorative Neurology and Neuroscience*, Vol. 35, No. 6, 2017, pp. 643–666.

Transforming Research and Clinical Knowledge in TBI, homepage, undated. As of November 29, 2021:
https://tracktbi.ucsf.edu/

Translational Research Center for TBI and Stress Disorders, homepage, November 30, 2021. As of December 28, 2021:
https://www.va.gov/boston-health-care/research/
the-translational-research-center-for-tbi-and-stress-disorders-tracts/

Traumatic Brain Injury Center of Excellence, *2020 Annual Report*, Falls Church, Va.: Military Health System, 2021.

Turner, G. M., C. McMullan, O. L. Aiyegbusi, D. Bem, T. Marshall, M. Calvert, J. Mant, and A. Belli, "Stroke Risk Following Traumatic Brain Injury: Systematic Review and Meta-Analysis," *International Journal of Stroke*, Vol. 16, No. 4, June 2021, pp. 370–384.

U.S. Department of Veterans Affairs, "Polytrauma System of Care Facilities," webpage, undated-a. As of August 30, 2021:
https://www.polytrauma.va.gov/system-of-care/care-facilities/index.asp

———, "Million Veteran Program (MVP): About," webpage, undated-b. As of December 2, 2021:
https://www.research.va.gov/mvp/

———, "Polytrauma/TBI System of Care: Rehabilitation Team," webpage, undated-c. As of August 30, 2021:
https://www.polytrauma.va.gov/about/Rehabilitation_Team.asp

———, *Assisted Living Pilot Program for Veterans with Traumatic Brain Injury (AL-TBI): July 1, 2017 to September 30, 2017, Quarterly and Final Report*, Washington, D.C., January 2018.

———, "Traumatic Brain Injury – Residential Rehabilitation (TBI-RR)," webpage, June 17, 2021. As of November 29, 2021:
https://www.va.gov/geriatrics/pages/
Traumatic_Brain_Injury_Residential_Rehabilitation_TBI_RR.asp

U.S Department of Veterans Affairs and U.S. Department of Defense, *VA/DoD Clinical Practice Guideline for the Management and Rehabilitation of Post-Acute Mild Traumatic Brain Injury*, Washington, D.C., 2021.

U. S. Food and Drug Administration, "Hyperbaric Oxygen Therapy: Don't Be Misled," FDA Consumer Health Information, August 2013, pp. 1–2.

———, "Hyperbaric Oxygen Therapy: Get the Facts," FDA Consumer Updates, July 26, 2021.

U.S. House of Representatives, *William H. (Mac) Thornberry National Defense Authorization Act for Fiscal Year 2021: Conference Report*, Washington, D.C., December 3, 2020.

VA—*See* U.S. Department of Veterans Affairs.

VA and DoD—*See* U.S. Department of Veterans Affairs and U.S. Department of Defense.

Vakil, E., Y. Greenstein, I. Weiss, and S. Shtein, "The Effects of Moderate-to-Severe Traumatic Brain Injury on Episodic Memory: A Meta-Analysis," *Neuropsychology Review*, Vol. 29, No. 3, September 2019, pp. 270–287.

Van Praag, D. L. G., M. C. Cnossen, S. Polinder, L. Wilson, and A. I. R. Maas, "Post-Traumatic Stress Disorder After Civilian Traumatic Brain Injury: A Systematic Review and Meta-Analysis of Prevalence Rates," *Journal of Neurotrauma*, Vol. 36, No. 23, December 2019, pp. 3220–3232.

Vanderbeken, I., and E. Kerckhofs, "A Systematic Review of the Effect of Physical Exercise on Cognition in Stroke and Traumatic Brain Injury Patients," *NeuroRehabilitation*, Vol. 40, No. 1, 2017, pp. 33–48.

VanderVeen, J. D., "TBI as a Risk Factor for Substance Use Behaviors: A Meta-Analysis," *Archives of Physical Medicine and Rehabilitation*, Vol. 102, No. 6, June 2021, pp. 1198–1209.

Virk, S., T. Williams, R. Brunsdon, F. Suh, and A. Morrow, "Cognitive Remediation of Attention Deficits Following Acquired Brain Injury: A Systematic Review and Meta-Analysis," *NeuroRehabilitation*, Vol. 36, No. 3, 2015, pp. 367–377.

Voinescu, A., J. Sui, and D. S. Fraser, "Virtual Reality in Neurorehabilitation: An Umbrella Review of Meta-Analyses," *Journal of Clinical Medicine*, Vol. 10, No. 7, April 2, 2021, article 1478.

Vos, B. C., K. Nieuwenhuijsen, and J. K. Sluiter, "Consequences of Traumatic Brain Injury in Professional American Football Players: A Systematic Review of the Literature," *Clinical Journal of Sport Medicine*, Vol. 28, No. 2, March 2018, pp. 91–99.

Warden, Deborah, "Military TBI During the Iraq and Afghanistan Wars," *Journal of Head Trauma Rehabilitation*, Vol. 21, No. 5, September–October 2006, pp. 398–402.

Warren, Sharon A., Susan Armijo Olivo, Jorge Fuentes Contreras, Karen V. L. Turpin, Douglas P. Gross, Linda J. Carroll, and Kenneth G. Warren, "Traumatic Injury and Multiple Sclerosis: A Systematic Review and Meta-Analysis," *Canadian Journal of Neurological Sciences*, Vol. 40, No. 2, 2013, pp. 168–176.

Watabe, T., H. Suzuki, M. Abe, S. Sasaki, J. Nagashima, and N. Kawate, "Systematic Review of Visual Rehabilitation Interventions for Oculomotor Deficits in Patients with Brain Injury," *Brain Injury*, Vol. 33, No. 13–14, 2019, pp. 1592–1596.

Watanabe, T. K., K. R. Bell, W. C. Walker, and K. Schomer, "Systematic Review of Interventions for Post-Traumatic Headache," *PM & R*, Vol. 4, No. 2, February 2012, pp. 129–140.

Watanabe, Y., and T. Watanabe, "Meta-Analytic Evaluation of the Association Between Head Injury and Risk of Amyotrophic Lateral Sclerosis," *European Journal of Epidemiology*, Vol. 32, No. 10, October 2017, pp. 867–879.

Weathers, F. W., B. T. Litz, T. M. Keane, P. A. Palmieri, B. P. Marx, and P. P. Schnurr, "The PTSD Checklist for DSM-5 (PCL-5)," webpage, 2013. As of October 20, 2021: https://www.ptsd.va.gov/professional/assessment/adult-sr/ptsd-checklist.asp

Weil, Z. M., J. D. Corrigan, and K. Karelina, "Alcohol Use Disorder and Traumatic Brain Injury," *Alcohol Research*, Vol. 39, No. 2, 2018, pp. 171–180.

Wheaton, P., J. L. Mathias, and R. Vink, "Impact of Pharmacological Treatments on Cognitive and Behavioral Outcome in the Postacute Stages of Adult Traumatic Brain Injury: A Meta-Analysis," *Journal of Clinical Psychopharmacology*, Vol. 31, No. 6, December 2011, pp. 745–757.

Wheeler, S., A. Acord-Vira, and D. Davis, "Effectiveness of Interventions to Improve Occupational Performance for People with Psychosocial, Behavioral, and Emotional Impairments After Brain Injury: A Systematic Review," *American Journal of Occupational Therapy*, Vol. 70, No. 3, May–June 2016.

Wiart, L., J. Luauté, A. Stefan, D. Plantier, and J. Hamonet, "Non Pharmacological Treatments for Psychological and Behavioural Disorders Following Traumatic Brain Injury (TBI). A Systematic Literature Review and Expert Opinion Leading to Recommendations," *Annals of Physical and Rehabilitation Medicine*, Vol. 59, No. 1, February 2016, pp. 31–41.

Wilk, J. E., R. K. Herrell, G. H. Wynn, L. A. Riviere, and C. W. Hoge, "Mild Traumatic Brain Injury (Concussion), Posttraumatic Stress Disorder, and Depression in U.S. Soldiers Involved in Combat Deployments: Association with Postdeployment Symptoms," *Psychosomatic Medicine*, Vol. 74, No. 3, April 2012, pp. 249–257.

Wilson, C. D., J. D. Burks, R. B. Rodgers, R. M. Evans, A. A. Bakare, and S. Safavi-Abbasi, "Early and Late Posttraumatic Epilepsy in the Setting of Traumatic Brain Injury: A Meta-Analysis and Review of Antiepileptic Management," *World Neurosurgery*, Vol. 110, February 2018, pp. E901–E906.

Wilson, S. H., M. Roth, A. S. Lindblad, and L. K. Weaver, "Review of Recent Non-Hyperbaric Oxygen Interventions for Mild Traumatic Brain Injury," *Undersea and Hyperbaric Medicine*, Vol. 43, No. 5, August–September 2016, pp. 615–627.

Winkens, I., C. M. Van Heugten, L. Fasotti, and D. T. Wade, "Treatment of Mental Slowness: How to Evaluate Treatment Effects. A Systematic Review of Outcome Measures," *Neuropsychological Rehabilitation*, Vol. 21, No. 6, December 2011, pp. 860–883.

Wobma, R., R. H. Nijland, J. C. Ket, and G. Kwakkel, "Evidence for Peer Support in Rehabilitation for Individuals with Acquired Brain Injury: A Systematic Review," *Journal of Rehabilitation Medicine*, Vol. 48, No. 10, November 2016, pp. 837–840.

Writer, Brian W., and Jason E. Schillerstrom, "Psychopharmacological Treatment for Cognitive Impairment in Survivors of Traumatic Brain Injury: A Critical Review," *Journal of Neuropsychiatry and Clinical Neurosciences*, Vol. 21, No. 4, Fall 2009, pp. 362–370.

Xu, G. Z., Y. F. Li, M. D. Wang, and D. Y. Cao, "Complementary and Alternative Interventions for Fatigue Management After Traumatic Brain Injury: A Systematic Review," *Therapeutic Advances in Neurological Disorders*, Vol. 10, No. 5, May 2017, pp. 229–239.

Ylvisaker, Mark, Lyn Turkstra, Carl Coehlo, Kathy Yorkston, Mary Kennedy, McKay Moore Sohlberg, and Jack Avery, "Behavioral Interventions for Children and Adults with Behaviour Disorders After TBI: A Systematic Review of the Evidence," *Brain Injury*, Vol. 21, No. 8, July 2007, pp. 769–805.

Yu, Z. Z., S. J. Jiang, Z. S. Jia, H. Y. Xiao, and M. Q. Zhou, "Study on Language Rehabilitation for Aphasia," *Chinese Medical Journal* (English ed.), Vol. 130, No. 12, June 2017, pp. 1491–1497.

Zhang, Y., Y. Ma, S. Chen, X. Liu, H. J. Kang, S. Nelson, and S. Bell, "Long-Term Cognitive Performance of Retired Athletes with Sport-Related Concussion: A Systematic Review and Meta-Analysis," *Brain Sciences*, Vol. 9, No. 8, August 13, 2019, article 199.

Zhao, L., Y. P. Wu, J. L. Qi, Y. Q. Liu, K. Zhang, and W. L. Li, "Efficacy of Levetiracetam Compared with Phenytoin in Prevention of Seizures in Brain Injured Patients: A Meta-Analysis," *Medicine*, Vol. 97, No. 48, November 2018, article e13247.

Zhou, L., and B. Parmanto, "Reaching People with Disabilities in Underserved Areas Through Digital Interventions: Systematic Review," *Journal of Medical Internet Research*, Vol. 21, No. 10, October 25, 2019, article e12981.